THE WEEKNIGHT MEDITERRANEAN KITCHEN

80 AUTHENTIC, HEALTHY RECIPES MADE QUICK AND EASY FOR EVERYDAY COOKING

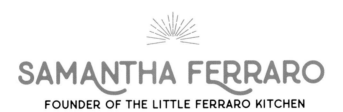

SAMANTHA FERRARO

FOUNDER OF THE LITTLE FERRARO KITCHEN

PAGE STREET
PUBLISHING CO.

PAGE STREET
PUBLISHING CO.

First published in 2018 by
Page Street Publishing Co.
27 Congress Street, Suite 105
Salem, MA 01970
www.pagestreetpublishing.com

Distributed by Macmillan, sales in Canada by The Canadian Manda Group.

22   21   20   19   18   1   2   3   4   5

ISBN-13: 978-1-62414-554-4
ISBN-10: 1-62414-554-X

Library of Congress Control Number: 2018930272

Cover and book design by Page Street Publishing Co.
Photography by Samantha Ferraro

Printed and bound in China

CONTENTS

CHAPTER 5
SAUCES, DIPS AND SPREADS
AROMATIC CONDIMENTS TO ENHANCE ANY DISH

143

CHAPTER 6
SWEETS AND SIPS
LIGHT AND FRUITY TREATS TO SATISFY YOUR SWEET TOOTH

169

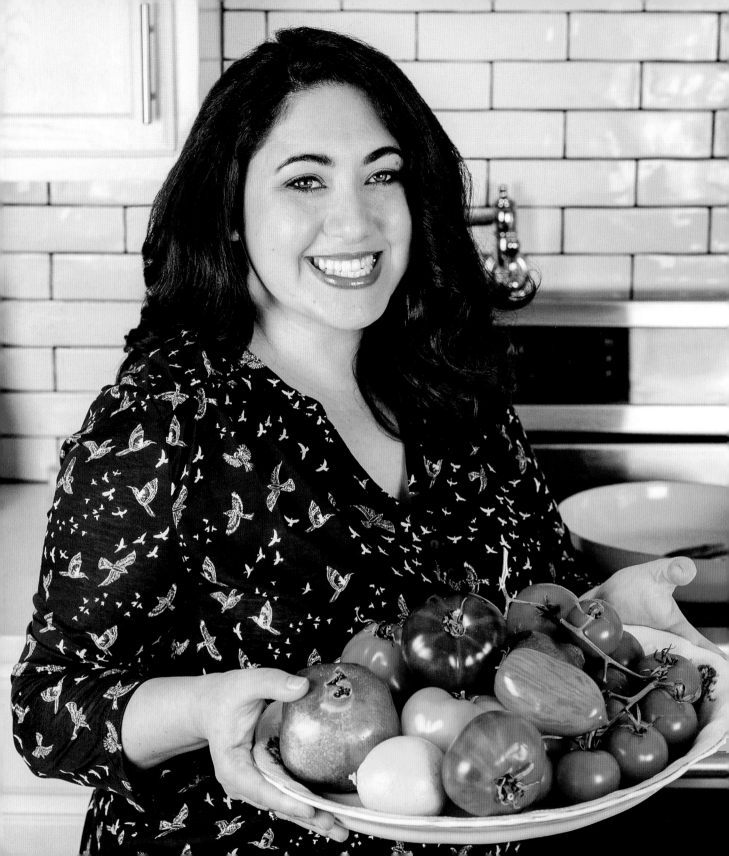

INTRODUCTION

I am still in shock as I am writing the introduction to this book. But when life hands you an opportunity, you run with it and make lemonade. Or muddled mint lemonade (check out the desserts chapter)! I've been blogging for the last four years or so, and, like other food bloggers, I love food; that goes without saying. But it's more than that. Cooking is not only about the food or the ingredients or standing in front of a stove and stirring. It's about the experience, the ultimate joy and passion you have for something you've created, spent time making and shared with yourself and with those you are feeding.

I come from a varied cultural background, and if you follow my blog, you know how much I appreciate and welcome learning about different cultures, including my own, through food. I have fond memories of my grandmother rolling cookie dough to make my favorite Jewish cookies called rugelach, and I can still smell the stems of her Jersey tomato plants. I wish I had taken that opportunity and learned from her, but it was years after she left us that I really appreciated what a good cook she was.

I have family on both sides of the Jewish world, which, let me tell you, I am soooo thankful for! My mom's side is Sephardic, with ancestry coming from Spain and Turkey. And my father's side is Ashkenazi, coming from Eastern Europe. I have been blessed to eat all sorts of Jewish foods growing up. Everything from pickled herring, to borscht, to yes—even gefilte fish! My mom had me rolling grape leaves stuffed with meat and rice as soon as I was walking. Eating dishes such as baba ganoush, creamy hummus and Turkish green bean stew called fasulye was the norm on a weeknight.

My thirtieth birthday was one I will never forget. That year, I graduated from college and ran a mini-triathlon, and my husband and I took the most exciting, life-changing trip to Turkey and Spain. It was that trip that truly connected me to my culture and heritage, and I am forever grateful. The food was diverse, seasonal and fresh, and it was at that moment when I thought, this is what cooking is all about.

Mediterranean food is my favorite to cook and eat. The food is simple and honest and made impressive with bold, flavorful spices such as smoked paprika, sumac and za'atar. People who eat a Mediterranean style diet have been known to live the longest lives by filling their plates with lean proteins, heart-healthy olive oil and loads of fresh seasonal produce.

The recipes in this book are a compilation of the flavors I love from ethnicities I admire. Some are traditional and some are my own interpretation of Mediterranean flavors and dishes. Mediterranean cuisine spans several continents and ethnicities. However, in this book I have focused on influences from my background, my upbringing and my travels. Turkey, Spain, Syria, Lebanon, Israel and Iran are just a few of the places that influenced these flavors and ultimately brought these recipes to life.

Cooking is an art, but it doesn't have to be time-consuming. Aromatic, flavor-punched meals should and can be enjoyed every day of the week—not just on weekends when you have more time. There is no perfect recipe, and there are always variables with everything you make. Use the best ingredients that you can afford and that are available to you, and don't be afraid to try something new.

My wish for you is to be inspired and ambitious. There are a lot of spices and flavors that are not as common as others, but what I hope is that you take these flavors and become excited and inquisitive, and that you try new recipes and experience new cultures.

MEDITERRANEAN PANTRY STAPLES

It's been said that if you have a well-stocked pantry you can make any dish within a minute's notice, or maybe that's just what I've always thought. And with that being said, all you need is a handful of flavorful spices and good-quality ingredients, and any dish can be prepared without much of a detailed recipe or deep thought.

My biggest premise when cooking the Mediterranean way is to be as fresh, seasonal and simple as possible. When you work with good-quality ingredients, you don't need to fuss much over anything else because the ingredients naturally shine, especially when complemented with added spices and flavors.

Here I'll share what we keep in our kitchen to help create easy, healthy weeknight meals.

LENTILS, RICE, COUSCOUS AND MORE

I raid my local store's bulk bin and buy only as much as I need. Lentils, rice, couscous, farro and orzo are all quick and easy to prepare and can mostly be used interchangeably. As I mention later on, hummus purists swear by dried beans, which I do keep in my pantry as well; however, on a weeknight when I'm tired, canned beans do just the trick. You can add beans to any dish like soups and salads for added texture and heartiness, or roast them for a simple snack.

FRESH HERBS

It goes without saying that we use a lot of herbs in our cooking. So much so that my overflowing mint plant (which grows quickly and easily) was nearly naked by the time I was done recipe testing. Mint and basil can often be used interchangeably. If you are not a fan of cilantro, use parsley instead—though I love the bright flavor of cilantro. Most of these recipes use the leaves only, so remove any thick stems or branches before pureeing or sautéing.

Storing fresh herbs is important, and you can extend freshness with a little extra care. Trim the ends and place the stems of a bunch of parsley or cilantro into a cup of shallow water.

Cover the whole cup with a resealable plastic bag, place in the fridge and change the water frequently. The leaves love the cool atmosphere and will stay fresh for at least a week. For fresh mint, dill and thyme, wrap in a slightly damp paper towel and store in the fridge. Basil, on the other hand, prefers a warmer environment, so store a bunch of basil in a shallow cup of water at room temperature.

OILS

Good-quality olive oil has amazing heart benefits and good-for-you fats. I often use regular olive oil when cooking and save the aromatic extra virgin olive oil for salad dressings or for a drizzle to finish the dish. For frying, however, I often lean towards grape-seed oil, which has a very mild flavor and can handle the high heat.

POMEGRANATE MOLASSES

A very thick and condensed syrup made by reducing pomegranate juice, pomegranate molasses has a tart and slightly sweet flavor to it. Because of its recent popularity, you can find pomegranate molasses at specialty stores and online. You can use pomegranate molasses to flavor salad dressings, as a marinade for lamb or as a drizzle on creamy tahini.

If pomegranate molasses is hard to find, try substituting with reduced balsamic vinegar. It won't be as tart but will still offer a very similar flavor profile.

TAHINI

Also called tahin, tahini is a paste made from ground sesame seeds. I have noticed different textures between certain brands and much prefer the creamier consistency. You can use tahini paste in a number of ways, such as in baked goods, whisked into a salad dressing, as a dipping sauce with lemon and garlic or simply spread on toast, and as the Israelis like it, with a drizzle of pomegranate molasses on top.

CITRUS

Lemon zest and juice are widely used throughout this book. Use a grater or microplane to grate the outside of the citrus, but don't grate all the way to the white pith, which can be bitter. Zest directly over the plate or bowl you're using to make the recipe so all the citrus oils can go directly into the dish. Citrus juice, on the other hand, has a different flavor profile than the zest and is more pungent and direct. Use citrus juice in salad dressings or as a finishing touch to your dish.

CHEESES AND YOGURT

Dairy ingredients have a strong presence in Mediterranean cuisine. Parmesan cheese is often used in Sephardic cooking and will make its appearance in a few dishes here and there. Feta cheese and halloumi cheese are also quite popular. Feta is popular in Greek cuisine and has a tangy, slightly briny flavor. Halloumi can be used to substitute for feta or vice versa; however, it has a bit more body to it and is not as salty as feta, so it can hold up to higher cooking temperatures during grilling or baking. Mediterraneans love their yogurts, as well. Most of these recipes call for thick, full-fat Greek yogurt, which in my opinion has the best flavor. If you prefer a thinner consistency, use regular full-fat yogurt. Fat-free yogurt will not offer the same texture or flavor intended in these recipes.

LEAN PROTEINS

Good-quality lean proteins are a very important aspect of creating healthy and quick meals. Mediterranean cooks use local proteins that are available within their region. Lamb is a popular protein found in dishes from Syria, Lebanon and Greece and is flavorful enough to be stuffed in tomatoes, marinated in yogurt for kabobs or grilled.

Try to buy the best quality meats and proteins you can afford, such as organic, free-range chicken and eggs and grass-fed beef and lamb.

Seafood, including shellfish, also is a good source of protein, and some shellfish like mussels and shrimp are inexpensive and can be cooked within minutes in a quick sauté of olive oil, garlic and chopped tomatoes. Mild white fish such as halibut or bass has a beautiful delicate flavor and soaks up aromatics when poached or sautéed with fresh herbs or simmered in a flavorful tomato sauce.

THE SPICES

The beautiful thing about Mediterranean cooking—in addition to the incredibly fresh and vibrant produce, the healthy fats and the bright flavors—is the wonderful use of spices. Deep, citrusy, smoky and spicy flavors can transform the most basic dish into something truly memorable.

Most of these spices can be found at your local grocer, and the harder to find ones can be found at gourmet food shops, such as Whole Foods or other international markets. If all else fails, they are easily ordered online. Below I break down the flavor profiles of the spices used in this book, offer a few substitution ideas and list the recipes that use each one. Have fun with them. Be inspired, and don't be afraid to get spicy!

ALEPPO PEPPER

This bright red pepper flake is named after the city of Aleppo, Syria, and has a sort of fruity note with a moderate heat level. If more flavor than heat is what you are looking for, Aleppo will be the perfect chili to add to your dishes. Due to recent events, Aleppo pepper is not easily sourced, though you may find it at some specialty stores and international markets and online. The maras pepper from Turkey is very similar to the Aleppo pepper and would make a good substitute. If you can't find Aleppo pepper, you may substitute about half the quantity with standard red chili flakes, which have a lot more heat than Aleppo flakes.

- Beef and Pine Nut Phyllo Rolls (page 18)
- Breakfast Pitas with Lamb, Tomatoes and Feta (page 33)
- Heirloom Tomato Bruschetta with Labneh (page 21)
- Za'atar Chicken Skewers (page 65)
- Slow Cooker Beef Stew with Green Beans, Potatoes and Spices (page 66)
- Baked Orzo with Artichokes, Tomatoes and Halloumi (page 115)
- Unstuffed Grape Leaves (page 107)

ALLSPICE

This is one of those background flavors that makes you go, "Hmmm . . . what's in this?" and makes you feel all warm and fuzzy inside. Many people think it is a mixture of "all the spices," but it is just one spice made from the dried berries of the Pimenta dioica plant. Because allspice has complex notes of cinnamon, clove and ginger, it seems to taste like all those things. Usually used in small quantities as a background flavor, allspice produces a beautiful warm note to both sweet and savory dishes and complements other warm spices, such as cinnamon, beautifully.

- Savory Cheese-Filled Pastries with Spicy Tomato Herb Sauce (page 26)
- Beef and Pine Nut Phyllo Rolls (page 21)
- Everyday Chicken Shawarma (page 62)
- Autumn Squash Salad with Figs and Arugula (page 101)
- Cauliflower Rice Pilaf with Lentils, Fried Onions and Burst Tomatoes (page 140)
- Mini Baklava Bites (page 173)

CARDAMOM

Mostly used in the form of whole dried pods or ground seeds, cardamom has an alluring fragrant note and is used in both sweet and savory dishes. Part of the same family as ginger, cardamom is known to aid in digestion and is used to freshen breath and improve overall oral health. Turks also add cardamom to their coffee, giving it a deep warm and slightly perfumed quality. To use the dried green cardamom pods, gently smash them and steep the pods in syrup or another liquid. You can also use a mortar and pestle to make freshly ground cardamom. However, already-ground cardamom is used in most recipes in this book and is also easily found at your local store or online.

- Mini Baklava Bites (page 173)
- Baked Cardamom French Toast with Peaches and Orange Blossom (page 170)
- Saffron-Poached Pears with Cardamom Pods (page 177)

CINNAMON

Cinnamon is usually thought of during the fall season for pumpkin-spiced lattes and desserts. However, Mediterranean cuisine uses cinnamon in a different way; it's instead added to savory dishes to offer a rich, warm layer of flavor. Cinnamon pairs very well with fall produce, such as figs and root vegetables, and in Lebanese cuisine it is often added to savory meat dishes, such as beef and pine nut phyllo rolls. A little goes a long way, and you'll never want to use more than a teaspoon in most savory recipes.

- Slow Cooker Beef with Green Beans, Potatoes and Spices (page 66)
- Harissa-Roasted Butternut Squash with Dates (page 136)
- Cauliflower Rice Pilaf with Lentils, Fried Onions and Burst Tomatoes (page 140)
- Mini Baklava Bites (page 173)
- Saffron-Poached Pears with Cardamom Pods (page 177)

CUMIN

Warm, rich and addictive, cumin is one of the most popular spices in the world and is even mentioned in the Bible. Used in cuisines all over the world, it's just as versatile sprinkled on meats, rubbed on vegetables and used in creative spice blends.

- Easy Homemade Harissa Sauce (page 144)
- Beef and Pine Nut Phyllo Rolls (page 18)
- Spiced Baked Pita Chips (page 42)
- Everyday Chicken Shawarma (page 62)
- Stuffed Eggplant with Meat and Tahini (page 58)
- Yogurt-Marinated Lamb and Eggplant Kabobs (page 54)
- Shakshuka with Lamb and Spices (page 46)
- Stuffed Tomatoes with Lamb and Feta (page 53)
- Cumin-Scented Squash and Lentil Soup with Crispy Chickpeas (page 81)
- Red Lentil Falafel (page 111)

GARLIC POWDER

Probably my most-used spice from the spice drawer—quite frankly, I use garlic powder whenever I am too lazy to chop up a few cloves. I probably wouldn't recommend using it to garnish, as it should cook down to really develop its flavor. If you want to use garlic as a final note, such as in bruschetta, then by all means take the time and chop up fresh garlic.

- Pita Nachos with Fried Eggplant and All the Toppings (page 39)
- Spiced Baked Pita Chips (page 42)
- Chopped Rainbow Salad with Crispy Lavash (page 98)
- Harissa Roasted Butternut Squash with Dates (page 136)

SAFFRON

Possibly one of the most intriguing spices of the world, saffron is the jewel of the spice world, as I like to say, and the most expensive, as well. Saffron is harvested from the crocus flower, making it incredibly rare and unique. Even though it takes many crocus flowers to produce an ounce (28 g) of saffron, you won't need more than a small pinch for most recipes. The flavor and color that saffron imparts is striking to say the least. The flavor and aroma are floral and earthy, and when steeped into water should produce a light yellow hue, which stains dishes (and your fingertips) very well. You can use saffron in both sweet and savory dishes, and it pairs beautifully with sweet tomatoes and simple dishes such as rice.

To use saffron you can do a number of things. Take a small pinch and allow the saffron to bloom in a few tablespoons of warm water, and then use that as your flavor agent. You can also take the saffron threads and grind them into a fine powder using a mortar and pestle. I have also heard of people lightly toasting saffron by putting the threads in a small foil packet and toasting over a flame. Sometimes I simply add the threads directly to my dish, which still produces the same appealing effect.

I want to mention that if color is all you're looking for, turmeric is a wonderful substitute and a lot less expensive, though it does not have the same floral qualities as saffron.

- Saffron Shrimp with Tomatoes and Feta (page 70)

- Creamy Saffron Cauliflower Soup with Paprika Oil (page 85)

- Basmati Rice with Pistachios, Lima Beans and Dill (page 119)

- Persian Rice with Turmeric and Saffron (page 123)

- Farro Paella with Seafood and Chorizo (page 104)

- Saffron-Poached Pears with Cardamom Pods (page 177)

- Rose-Saffron Crème Brûlée (page 181)

SALT

I wanted to mention salt because I find it to be such a personal preference. The amounts of salt called for in the recipes should be a general guideline, but above all, it depends on your palate. The salt tested for these recipes and used in my home is almost always kosher salt. I never, ever use table salt, as I find it bitter and yes, too salty. Kosher salt is a bit coarser and has a lighter note. My other favorite salt is the Maldon brand of sea salt flakes that I use as a finishing salt. These salt flakes are light with an almost sweet-salty taste to them.

PAPRIKA

One of my favorite flavors, paprika is a ground spice made from dried peppers. Paprika ranges in flavor profile as well as heat, coming in both sweet and, my ultimate favorite, smoky varieties. Most of the recipes that include paprika in this book call for the smoked paprika version because I love those robust flavors. However, if that isn't to your liking as much, feel free to substitute with mild and sweet paprika, which will still offer the overall warm flavors and beautiful color.

- Breakfast Egg and Avocado Pastries with Harissa Salsa (page 30)

- One-Pot Paprika Chicken with Olives and Orzo (page 49)

- Everyday Chicken Shawarma (page 62)

- Shakshuka with Lamb and Spices (page 42)

- Stuffed Tomatoes with Lamb and Feta (page 53)

- Creamy Saffron Cauliflower Soup with Paprika Oil (page 85)

- Farro Paella with Seafood and Chorizo (page 104)

SUMAC

A sour, tart and citrusy spice, sumac is one of the distinctive ingredients in za'atar (mentioned a bit later). The berries of the sumac bush, which is native to the Middle East, are dried and ground to create sumac spice. A small dusting adds an amazing brightness to any dish. If sumac is difficult to find, you can substitute with some freshly grated lemon zest or a squeeze of lemon juice.

- Savory Cheese-Filled Pastries with Spicy Tomato Herb Sauce (page 26)
- Pita Nachos with Fried Eggplant and All the Toppings (page 39)
- Everyday Chicken Shawarma (page 62)
- Pomegranate-Glazed Lamb Chops (page 61)
- Shakshuka with Lamb and Spices (page 46)
- Roasted Pepper and Tomato Soup with Broiled Halloumi Cheese (page 74)
- Fennel Fattoush Salad with Pistachios (page 86)
- Summer Fruit and Heirloom Tomato Panzanella with Basil Mint Vinaigrette (page 90)
- Turkish Eggs with Spinach and Yogurt (page 127)
- Broccoli Rabe with Chickpeas and Garlic Pine Nuts (page 139)

TURMERIC

Also known as the "poor man's saffron," turmeric use has been dated back nearly 4,000 years. Used to color clothing, makeup and of course food, turmeric is used all over the world for its amazing anti-inflammatory properties. With a deep earthy flavor and an exotic golden hue, turmeric can be added to just about any dish, including soups, vegetables and even drinks, or as a spice rub for proteins. You can use a microplane or grater to grate the fresh root. Just make sure to either clean the tool immediately after use or designate a grater just for the turmeric, as it will stain anything it touches. Ground dried turmeric is also easily found in stores and can be added as you would fresh. In these recipes, ground dried turmeric is used.

- Everyday Chicken Shawarma (page 62)
- Olive Oil-Braised Chicken with Fennel and Citrus (page 57)
- Yogurt-Marinated Lamb and Eggplant Kabobs (page 54)
- Cumin-Scented Squash and Lentil Soup with Crispy Chickpeas (page 81)
- Chopped Salad with Farro, Crispy Chickpeas and Turmeric Vinaigrette (page 94)
- Red Lentil Falafel (page 111)

ZA'ATAR

This blend of spices includes a mixture of thyme, oregano, sumac and sesame, though there are different varieties available. Za'atar has an addictive and earthy flavor and is versatile enough to garnish dishes, sprinkle on breads, marinate meats or be added to roasted vegetables or salad dressings. To be honest, it's hard to offer a substitution for za'atar, so do your best hunting it down. Because of its recent popularity, you can most likely find za'atar at many grocery stores, specialty markets and definitely online. Some of my favorite brands are Sadaf and The Spice Hut.

- Tahini Toasts, Any Way You Like It (page 29)
- Grilled Za'atar-Spiced Flatbread with Squash Blossoms (page 38)
- Spiced Baked Pita Chips (page 42)
- Za'atar Chicken Skewers (page 65)
- Stuffed Tomatoes with Lamb and Feta (page 53)
- Beet-Infused Israeli Couscous with Beet Vinaigrette (page 116)
- Mediterranean Ratatouille with Pistachio Pesto (page 128)

TIP: If you can't find za'atar, making the spice blend couldn't be easier. Mix a batch and keep it in a small glass jar for easy use. To make ¾ cup (57 g) of za'atar spice blend, combine 2 tablespoons (6 g) of dried thyme, 2 tablespoons (28 g) of sumac, 2 tablespoons (16 g) of toasted sesame seeds, 1 tablespoon (6 g) of dried oregano and ¼ teaspoon of salt.

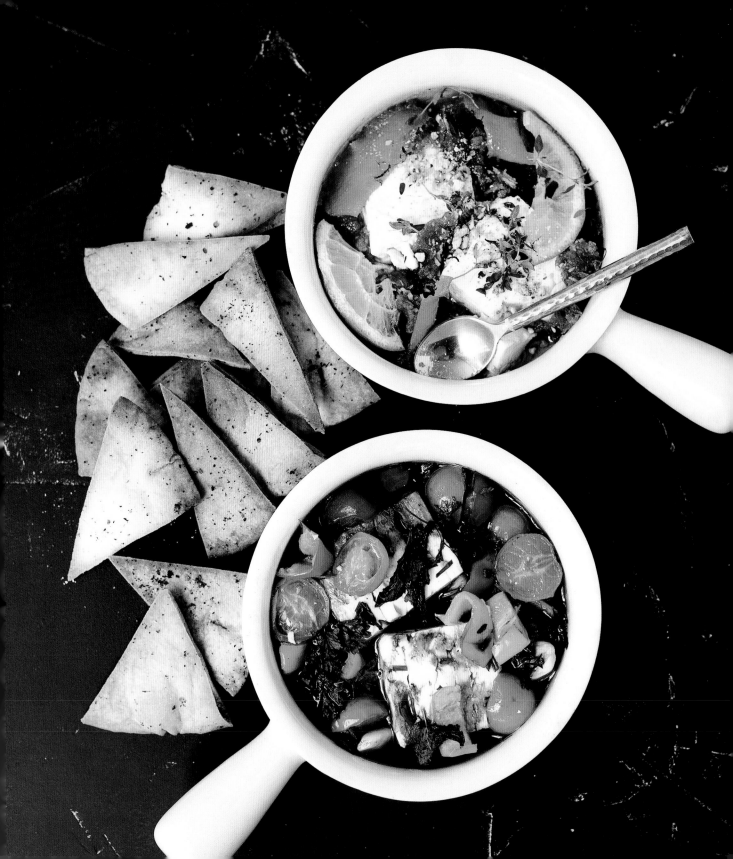

CHAPTER 1

APPETIZERS AND MEZZE

FAST AND FRESH LIGHT FARE

It wasn't until my husband and I visited Turkey and Spain a few years back that we really appreciated mezze and tapas. Mezze and tapas are small plates of appetizers with different textures and flavors, each one more exciting and interesting than the last. Some examples are petite bites of bruschetta, cheese, olives and savory pastry pockets called bourekas. All can be enjoyed as a quick mezze or as part of a Mediterranean breakfast.

I will never forget the times we stood at bars in Spain in front of rows and rows of different small plates. Crostini topped with tomatoes and small bowls filled with fresh seafood were some of my favorite eats.

All of these memories and flavors inspired the recipes in this chapter and are perfect for the quick last-minute get-together or afternoon snack.

Spiced Baked Pita Chips (page 42) with deep aromatic spices are crunchy and addictive. Add them to salads or make a batch for a quick snack. Savory Cheese-Filled Pastries with Spicy Tomato Herb Sauce (page 26) are eaten at breakfast in Turkey or can be made ahead of time and easily reheated for a weekday lunch. If you have some last-minute guests and need a quick appetizer, Citrus-Roasted Olives and Artichoke Hearts (page 25) are easy to prepare with minimal prep time and are always a crowd pleaser.

BEEF AND PINE NUT PHYLLO ROLLS

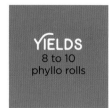

When my husband and I were traveling in Turkey, we ate our weight in their popular savory pastries known as bourekas or boreks. They come in an array of shapes and sizes—some layered and cut into squares or boreks folded into little pockets like the Savory Cheese Pastries on page 26. But it was the cigar-shaped bourekas that intrigued us the most due to their unique and fun shape. Serve them as a quick appetizer or small bite and dip them into Magical Herb Tahini Sauce (page 147) or Mediterranean Green Romesco (page 151).

6 tbsp (90 ml) olive oil, divided

½ lb (226 g) ground beef

1 small shallot, chopped finely

2 garlic cloves, chopped finely

½ tsp ground cinnamon

½ tsp ground allspice

½ tsp ground cumin

¼ tsp ground pepper

1 tsp salt, divided

¼ cup (34 g) pine nuts

⅓ cup (10 g) loosely packed parsley leaves, chopped finely

½ package frozen phyllo dough, about 20 sheets, defrosted

1 tsp sesame seeds, for topping

1 tsp Aleppo pepper flakes, for topping

TIP: The trick to working with phyllo is to be confident and forgiving. Some phyllo sheets will dry and break, but that is OK, and once they are rolled up no one will know the difference. As you are working with the phyllo, keep the unused pile covered with a damp towel so it won't dry out.

Preheat the oven to 375°F (190°C) and line a baking sheet with parchment paper.

In a medium-size skillet, over medium-high heat, add 2 tablespoons (30 ml) of the olive oil and the ground beef. Use a wooden spatula to break up the meat and cook until mostly cooked through, about 3 to 4 minutes.

Add the shallot and continue cooking for another 2 minutes. Add the garlic and cook for another minute, until both the shallot and garlic soften and turn a light golden color.

Stir in the cinnamon, allspice, cumin, pepper and ½ teaspoon salt, along with the pine nuts and parsley, and sauté everything together. Once the meat is fully cooked, taste for seasoning and adjust if needed. Turn off the heat and transfer the meat mixture to a bowl or plate to cool down for a few minutes.

Unroll the phyllo sheets and cut them in half horizontally, so you'll have two stacks of square sheets. Place a damp towel over them as you work to keep the sheets from getting dry.

Layer 4 to 5 phyllo sheets on a clean surface and spoon 1 to 2 tablespoons (15 to 30 g) of meat filling towards the bottom one-third of the phyllo. Brush the edges lightly with olive oil and roll up the phyllo, tucking in the ends about halfway through and rolling tightly until a long cigar shape forms. Continue with the rest of the sheets until you have used up all the filling.

Place the phyllo rolls on the baking sheet and brush the tops with the remaining olive oil.

Sprinkle the remaining salt, sesame seeds and Aleppo pepper all over the tops of the pastries, and bake for 15 minutes or until the pastries are lightly golden brown and crunchy on the outside.

Once done, allow to cool for a few minutes and serve with your favorite dip.

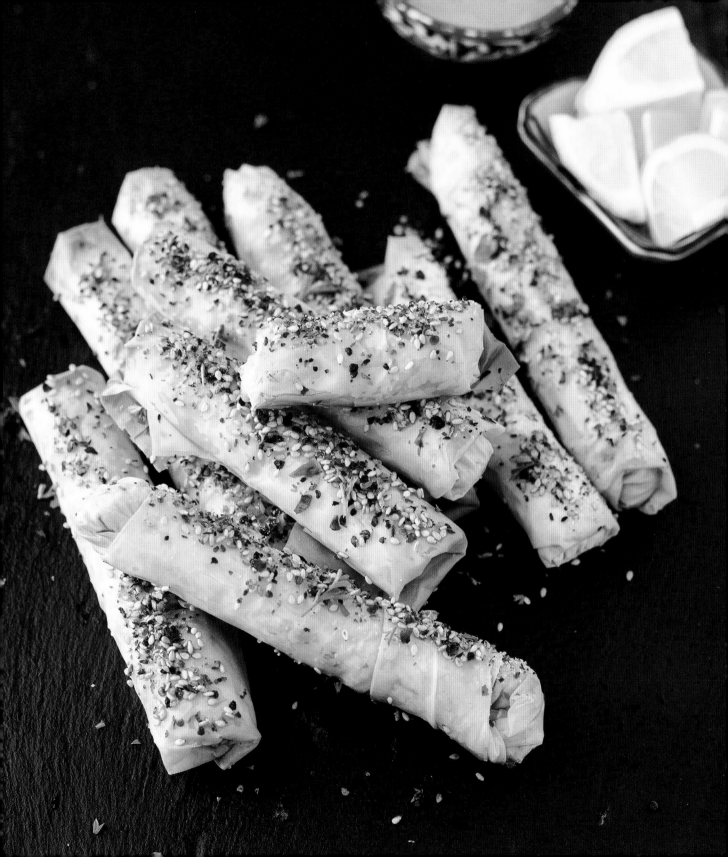

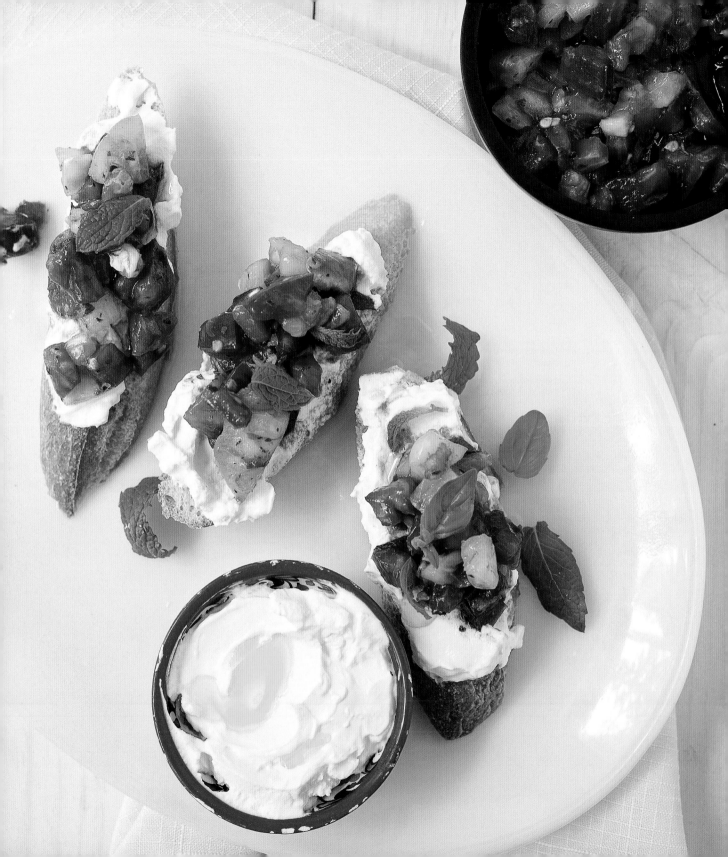

HEIRLOOM TOMATO BRUSCHETTA
WITH LABNEH

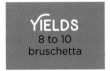

YIELDS
8 to 10
bruschetta

I can still smell the tomato vines from my grandmother's New Jersey tomato garden. Ever since then, tomatoes have been my candy. I eat them as often as the season allows and keep them as classic as can be. A simple and flavorful bruschetta is quick to pull together and teams up beautifully with tangy labneh cheese. If you can't find labneh, feel free to substitute full-fat Greek yogurt.

1 large baguette, cut into 10–12 diagonal slices

6 oz (170 g) labneh

3 medium-sized heirloom tomatoes, cut into ¼-inch (6-mm) pieces

2 garlic cloves, grated

¼ cup (5 g) fresh mint leaves, chopped finely, plus more for garnish

2 tbsp (30 ml) olive oil, plus more for garnish

1 tbsp (15 ml) balsamic vinegar

½ tsp salt

½ tsp Aleppo pepper flakes

Preheat the oven to 400°F (204°C) and arrange the baguette slices in a single layer on a baking sheet. Toast the slices for about 5 minutes until lightly golden brown. You can also grill the bread slices in a grill pan or over an outdoor grill.

Remove the bread from the oven and allow to cool for a few minutes. Spoon about 1 tablespoon (15 g) of labneh onto each baguette slice.

In a bowl, combine the tomatoes, garlic, mint, olive oil, vinegar, salt and Aleppo pepper and toss well to combine. Taste for seasoning and adjust as needed. Spoon the tomato mixture on top of the labneh.

Garnish the bruschetta with an extra drizzle of olive oil and fresh mint leaves.

TIP: When heirlooms aren't in season, feel free to use any deep red vine or roma tomatoes. Be sure to store them at room temperature with the stem side down for the best tasting tomatoes.

BAKED FETA TWO WAYS

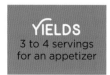

YIELDS
3 to 4 servings
for an appetizer

I couldn't resist sharing a recipe for both a sweet and savory cheese mezze. Feta is a wonderful base for flavorings and pairs beautifully with a touch of sweet honey and fresh herbs or with the classic flavors of tomato, garlic and oregano. Either way, this delectable cheese appetizer is done in nearly 20 minutes with minimal prep time. Serve with Spiced Baked Pita Chips (page 42) or fresh vegetables.

SAVORY BAKED FETA WITH TOMATO AND GARLIC

4 oz (113 g) block feta cheese

6 cherry tomatoes, cut in half

3 mini bell peppers, seeds removed and roughly chopped

2 garlic cloves, smashed

1 sprig oregano, stem removed

1 sprig mint leaves, stem removed

2 sprigs parsley, hard stems removed

3 tbsp (45 ml) olive oil

1 tbsp (15 ml) balsamic vinegar

SWEET BAKED FETA WITH HONEY AND THYME

4 oz (113 g) block feta cheese

3–4 sprigs thyme

3 tbsp (45 ml) olive oil

1 tbsp (15 ml) honey

3 strips orange zest

2 pitted dates, roughly chopped

SAVORY BAKED FETA WITH TOMATO AND GARLIC

Preheat the oven to 350°F (176°C) and add the feta, tomatoes, peppers, garlic, oregano, mint, parsley, oil and vinegar to a 6-inch (15-cm) oven-safe dish. Bake for 20 minutes, until the top of the cheese is a light golden color and the tomatoes have softened and released their juices. Remove from the oven and allow to cool for 5 minutes before serving.

SWEET BAKED FETA WITH HONEY AND THYME

Preheat the oven to 350°F (176°C) and add the feta, thyme, oil, honey, zest and dates to a 6-inch (15-cm) oven-safe dish. Bake for 20 minutes, until the top of the cheese is a light golden color and the honey has melted. Remove from the oven and allow to cool for 5 minutes before serving.

TIP: Use a vegetable peeler to peel strips of orange zest. The oils in the orange zest will add a deep sweet citrus flavor.

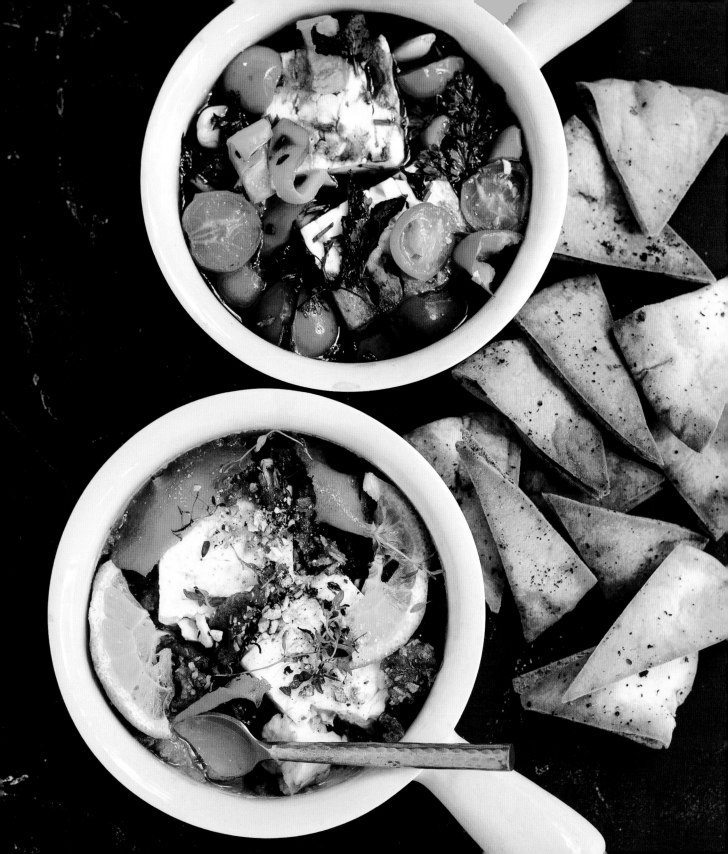

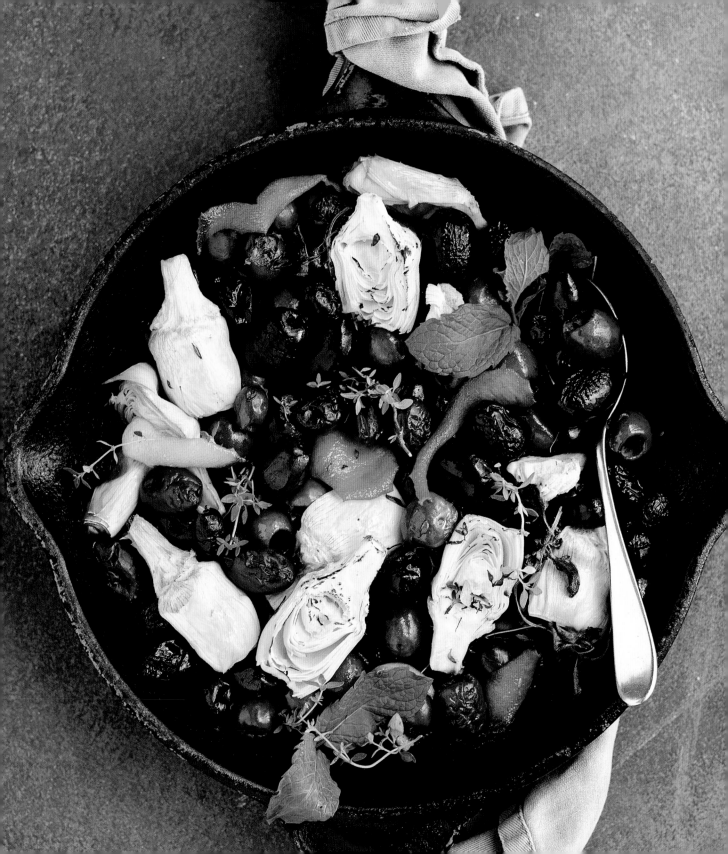

CITRUS-ROASTED OLIVES AND ARTICHOKE HEARTS

YIELDS
4 to 6 servings
for an appetizer

An appetizer could not get any simpler than this. Mixed olives are paired with strips of citrus peel that, when cooked enough, can be eaten entirely. Serve with Baked Feta Two Ways (page 22) and Za'atar Flatbread (page 38).

16 oz (453 g) assorted olives

15 oz (425 g) frozen and defrosted or canned artichoke hearts, cut in half

3–4 strips orange peel

3–4 strips lemon peel

Small bunch herbs, including thyme and oregano

Olive oil, as needed

Fresh oregano leaves, for garnish

Preheat the oven to 400°F (204°C) and arrange the olives, artichokes, citrus peels and herbs in an oven-safe dish or cast iron pan. Toss to combine and drizzle the top with olive oil.

Bake for 20 minutes until the citrus peels begin to caramelize and become aromatic. Serve immediately garnished with fresh oregano.

 TIP: Use a vegetable peeler to peel thin strips of citrus peel.

SAVORY CHEESE-FILLED PASTRIES
WITH SPICY TOMATO HERB SAUCE

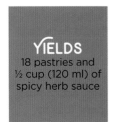

YIELDS
18 pastries and
½ cup (120 ml) of
spicy herb sauce

These savory pastries, called bourekas, are found in Turkey and all over Israel. You can find bourekas filled with everything from meats to eggplant to spinach and, my absolute favorite, cheese. Think of this as a savory hand pie of sorts; the vessel can be anything from puff pastry to phyllo. The spicy tomato herb sauce is a boureka's best friend. A fiery condiment called zhoug is full of fresh herbs, spicy chilies and, in my version, a sweet roasted tomato. My advice: Make extra sauce and slather it on grilled vegetables and meats. It will be your new favorite condiment. If fresh tomatoes aren't in season, feel free to substitute ¼ cup (14 g) of sundried tomatoes.

1 whole medium-sized tomato, cut in half and seeded

CHEESE PASTRIES

2 sheets puff pastry, thawed

1 cup (150 g) crumbled feta cheese

⅓ cup (28 g) shredded mozzarella cheese

2 eggs, divided

¼ tsp salt

Ground pepper

1 tbsp (15 ml) milk

2 tbsp (18 g) sesame seeds

1 tbsp (9 g) ground sumac

SPICY TOMATO HERB SAUCE

1 jalapeño (seeded, optional unless you prefer more heat)

½ cup (15 g) fresh cilantro, hard stems removed

½ cup (15 g) fresh parsley, hard stems removed

2 garlic cloves, roughly chopped

1 tsp ground cumin

½ tsp ground cardamom

¼ tsp ground allspice

1–2 tbsp (15–30 ml) olive oil

1–2 tbsp (15–30 ml) water

Salt, to taste

Place the tomato on a parchment-lined baking sheet and roast at 400°F (204°C) for 25 minutes or until softened and slightly charred. Once done, remove it from the oven and allow to cool. Reduce the temperature to 375°F (190°C) for the pastries.

Once the tomato is cool, remove the outer skin and roughly chop the flesh. Set aside.

For the pastries, unfold the thawed puff pastry sheets and gently roll out the pastry so it's a bit thinner to work with. Use a sharp knife and cut each sheet into 9 equal squares.

In a bowl, add both cheeses and 1 egg, season with salt and pepper and mix to combine.

Place a spoonful of the cheese mixture into the center of each pastry square and seal the edges, forming a triangle. If the pastry is a bit dry, use a wet finger to help seal the edges. Place all of the pastries on a parchment-lined baking sheet.

Whisk together the other egg and milk in a bowl and brush the egg wash onto all the pastries. Sprinkle sesame seeds and sumac on top and bake the bourekas at 375°F (190°C) for about 25 minutes, or until the pastry has puffed and the outside is a nice golden brown.

To make the spicy herb sauce, add the tomato, jalapeño, cilantro, parsley, garlic, cumin, cardamom, allspice, oil, water and salt to a food processor and pulse until it's finely chopped, but not overly pureed. It should be the consistency of a coarse chimichurri. Taste for seasoning and adjust the consistency as needed, adding a bit more water to help it get moving.

Serve the savory cheese pastries with the herb sauce on the side.

 TIP: Instead of roasting the tomato, you can grill it for a smokier flavor.

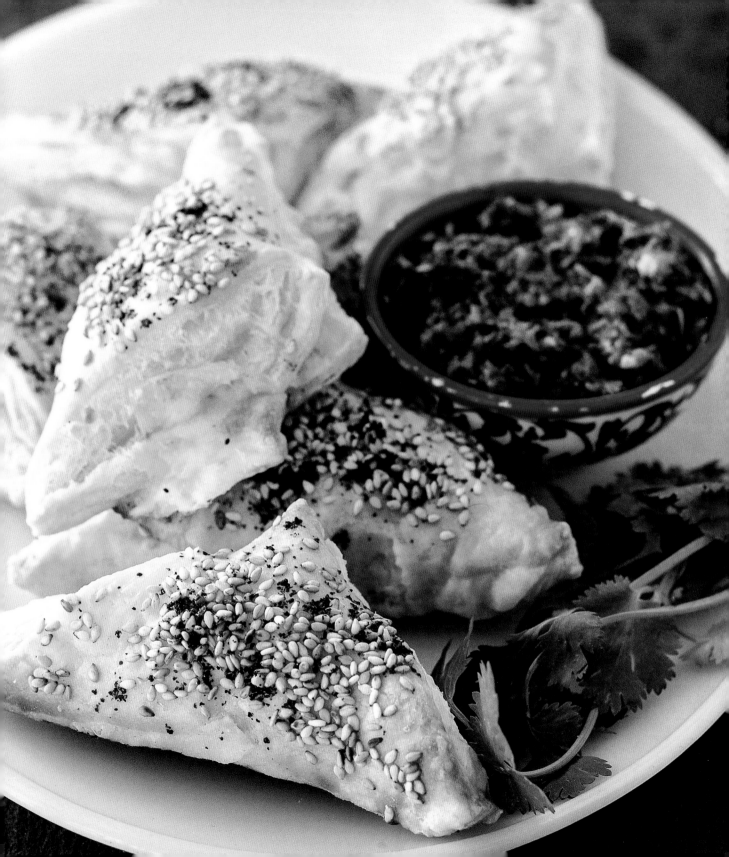

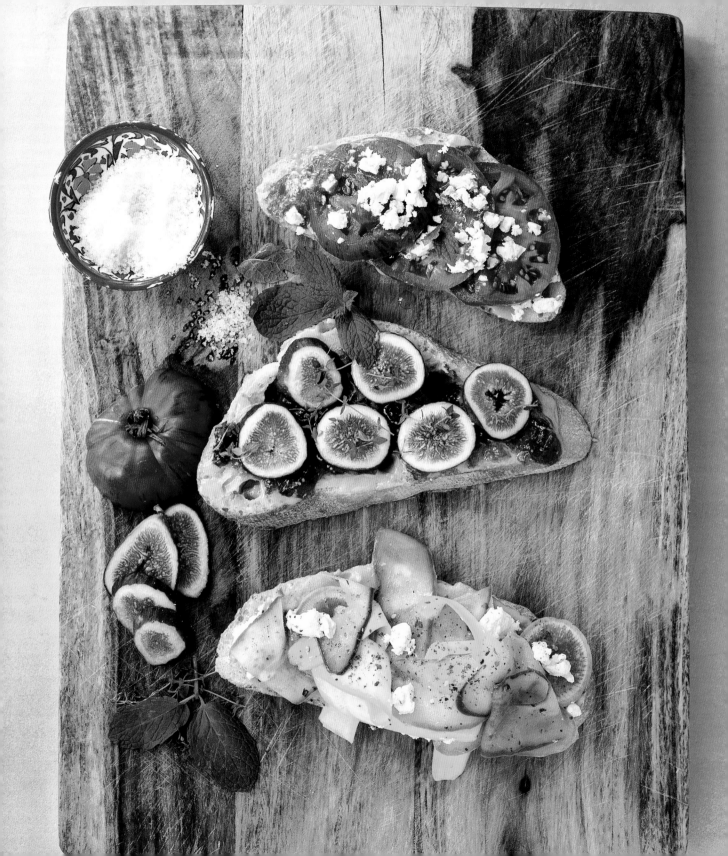

TAHINI TOASTS, ANYWAY YOU LIKE IT

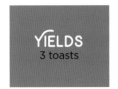

YIELDS
3 toasts

Step aside avocado toast, tahini toast is where it's at. A thick creamy spread made from ground sesame seeds, tahini has a deep nutty flavor and is loaded with protein to keep you fed, fueled and ready to take on the day.

Spread tahini on your favorite toasted bread and top with desired toppings. Here, I have both sweet and savory toasts for your inspiration—but really, just have fun with it.

3 slices of your favorite bread, toasted

SAVORY SPICY TAHINI TOAST

2 tbsp (30 ml) tahini

1 tbsp (15 ml) harissa

3 slices tomato

1 oz (28 g) crumbled feta cheese

Fresh mint leaves

Olive oil, for drizzling

SAVORY TAHINI TOAST WITH VEGETABLE RIBBONS, LEMON AND ZA'ATAR

1 small seedless cucumber, very thinly peeled

1 small zucchini, sliced very thinly using a vegetable peeler

1 tsp za'atar

1 tbsp (15 ml) lemon juice

1 tbsp (15 ml) olive oil

2 tbsp (30 ml) tahini

1 oz (28 g) goat cheese

Salt, to taste

SWEET TAHINI TOAST WITH FIG AND THYME

1 tbsp (15 ml) tahini

1 tbsp (15 ml) fig jam

2 figs, sliced thin

2 sprigs fresh thyme, leaves removed

SAVORY SPICY TAHINI TOAST

Spread the tahini on the toast and then top with the harissa. Lay the tomato slices on top and garnish with cheese, mint and a light drizzle of oil.

SAVORY TAHINI TOAST WITH VEGETABLE RIBBONS, LEMON AND ZA'ATAR

In a small bowl, toss together the cucumber and zucchini ribbons along with the za'atar, juice and oil. Spread the tahini on the toasted bread and layer the peeled vegetables on top. Crumble the goat cheese on the top and season with salt.

SWEET TAHINI TOAST WITH FIG AND THYME

Spread the tahini and fig jam on the toast. Lay the fig slices on top and garnish with fresh thyme leaves.

BREAKFAST EGG AND AVOCADO PASTRIES WITH HARISSA SALSA

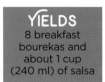

YIELDS
8 breakfast
bourekas and
about 1 cup
(240 ml) of salsa

There is nothing like a Mediterranean breakfast filled with cheeses, olives, fresh fruit and savory pastries like bourekas. I took inspiration from some of my favorite American breakfast flavors and folded them into a savory pastry to create a sort of mash-up of food cultures, if you will. The paired harissa salsa has all the flavors of common Easy Homemade Harissa Sauce (page 144), just chopped up a bit differently into a free-form salsa.

BREAKFAST PASTRIES

1 tbsp (15 g) butter

5 whole eggs, plus 1 egg for egg wash

1 tbsp (15 ml) milk

¼ tsp salt

Ground pepper

½ cup (75 g) crumbled feta cheese

2 sheets puff pastry, thawed

1 avocado, gently mashed

1 tsp za'atar

1 tsp sesame seeds

HARISSA SALSA

2 medium-sized tomatoes, chopped into ¼-inch (6-mm) pieces

1 roasted bell pepper, chopped into ¼-inch (6-mm) pieces

1 garlic clove, grated

1 lemon, juiced

½ tsp ground cumin

½ tsp paprika

¼ tsp salt, or more to taste

1 fresno or serrano pepper, chopped finely (seeds removed for less heat)

¼ cup (5 g) loosely packed cilantro leaves, hard stems removed and chopped finely

For the breakfast pastries, preheat the oven to 350°F (176°C) and line a baking sheet with parchment paper.

Melt the butter in a non-stick skillet over low-medium heat and whisk together the 5 eggs, milk, salt and pepper in a bowl. Pour the egg mixture into the pan and slowly scramble the eggs until gently cooked through, about 3 to 5 minutes. As soon as the eggs are almost done, add in the feta, turn off the heat and fold in. Once done, transfer to a plate and set aside.

Unroll the thawed puff pastry and use a rolling pin to gently roll the pastry a bit thinner. Cut each pastry sheet into four equal squares or 3-inch (7.6-cm) rounds and divide the egg mixture and mashed avocado among the squares.

Fold over the puff pastry, creating a hand pie, and crimp the edges with a fork. Use a small paring knife to cut a small slit on the top of each pastry.

Whisk the remaining egg and brush over the pastries. Sprinkle with za'atar and sesame seeds and bake for about 25 minutes or until the pastry has puffed up and is lightly golden brown. Allow them to cool slightly before handling.

To make the harissa salsa, add the tomatoes, bell pepper, garlic, lemon juice, cumin, paprika, salt, fresno pepper and cilantro to a bowl and mix thoroughly. For a saucier consistency, use the back of a spoon to gently mash the tomatoes. Serve alongside the pastries.

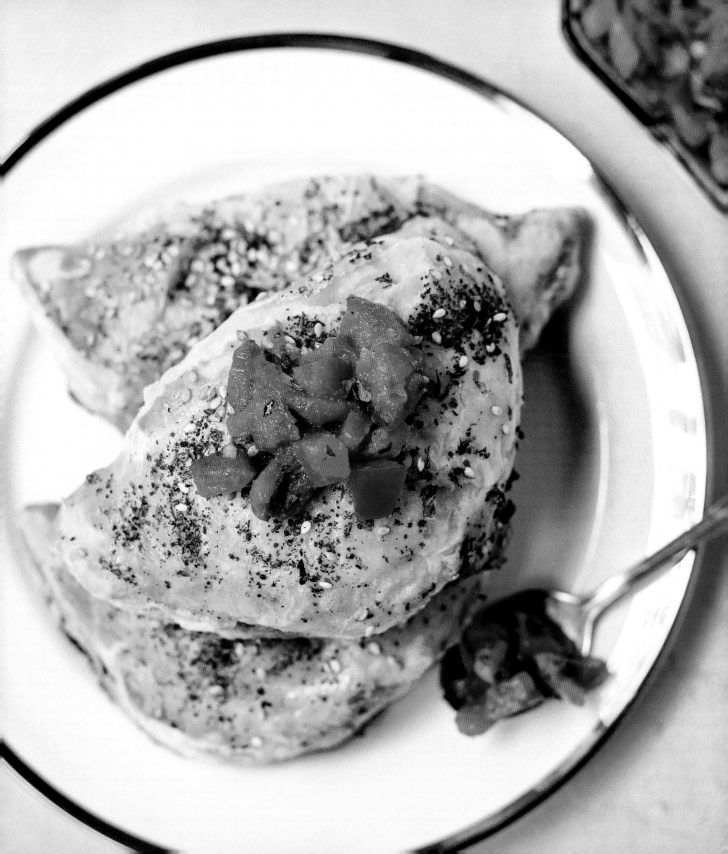

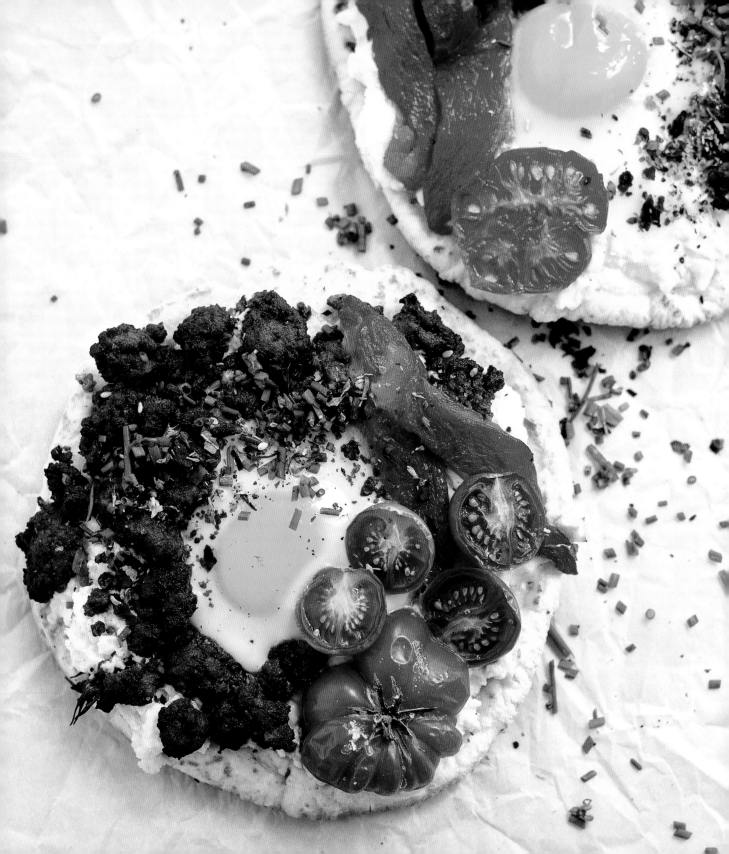

BREAKFAST PITAS WITH LAMB, TOMATOES AND FETA

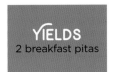

YIELDS
2 breakfast pitas

This recipe is a loose representation of a dish called pide, which is a traditional oval-shaped Turkish pizza filled with cheeses, meats and tomatoes cooked in an incredibly hot oven. The edges are crisp, the dough wafer-thin and the filling savory and hot. The classic dough takes time and yeast; because I like an easier dough, thick pitas are the perfect vessel to deliver the same robust flavors.

1 tsp olive oil

6 oz (170 g) ground lamb

1½ tsp (4 g) za'atar, divided

½ tsp ground cumin

Salt, as needed

Pepper, as needed

2 pita breads

4 tbsp (60 g) ricotta cheese

½ roasted bell pepper, cut in pieces

2 whole eggs

4 tbsp (60 g) feta cheese

4 cherry tomatoes, cut in half

1 tbsp (3 g) chopped chives

Aleppo pepper flakes, for garnish

Preheat the oven to 400°F (204°C).

Drizzle the olive oil into a small skillet and place on medium heat. Add the ground lamb and use a wooden spatula to break up the meat.

Add ½ teaspoon of za'atar, the cumin, salt and pepper and continue cooking until the lamb is cooked all the way through. Once done, reserve to a plate.

Lay the pita bread on a parchment-lined baking sheet and spread 2 tablespoons (30g) of ricotta on each pita, making a small well in the center to allow for the egg.

Divide both the ground lamb and roasted bell pepper pieces between the two pitas, scattering them along the edge, which will also help the egg stay in place.

Crack 2 whole eggs separately and add each one to the pitas, making sure they are somewhat centered. Sprinkle the feta cheese around both pitas and top with the cherry tomatoes.

Bake for 7 to 8 minutes until the egg whites are set. Garnish with chives, Aleppo pepper and reserved za'atar.

 TIP: This recipe is so versatile you can use any vegetables you have. Leftover Harissa-Roasted Butternut Squash with Dates (page 136) would work great in this, too!

STEAMED MUSSELS WITH TOMATO AND HARISSA

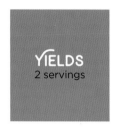

YIELDS
2 servings

When I was growing up on the East Coast, my grandparents would often take us out for mussels on special occasions. My cousins and I would fight over huge bowls filled with mussels and marinara, and later I realized how mandatory mussels were in Mediterranean cuisine as well. If you ever get a chance to walk the streets of Istanbul, you'll see piles of fresh black mussels in every corner, ready to be stuffed as the Turks do, or in this case, simply steamed. The beautiful thing about mussels is that they are mild, incredibly tender and ridiculously quick to prepare. The chopped tomatoes soften just enough for a little sweetness and the spicy harissa gives you just enough of a snappy bite.

3 tbsp (45 ml) olive oil

1 small shallot, sliced

3 garlic cloves, chopped finely

2 tbsp (30 ml) tomato paste

2 tbsp (30 ml) Easy Homemade Harissa Sauce (page 144)

1 medium-sized tomato, chopped into ½-inch (1.2-cm) pieces

¼ cup (60 ml) white wine

1 lb (453 g) mussels, washed and debearded

½ cup (10 g) chopped fresh parsley or basil

¼ tsp salt, or more as needed

Lemon wedges, for serving

Heat a medium-size skillet, anywhere from 10 to 13 inches (25 to 33 cm) wide over medium heat and drizzle with the olive oil. Add the shallot, sautéing until softened and lightly golden, about 2 to 3 minutes.

Add the garlic and sauté for another 1 to 2 minutes, and then stir in the tomato paste and harissa, making sure the paste melts into the oil.

Add the tomatoes and white wine, stirring until the tomatoes begin to release their juices and the wine reduces, another 1 to 2 minutes.

Add in the mussels and use a spatula to toss everything together. Cover the pan with a lid and cook until the mussels have opened, another 3 to 5 minutes. Throw away any mussels that have not opened.

Season with the parsley and salt and serve with the lemon wedges.

TIP: Be sure to clean your mussels before cooking them. Use a kitchen towel and pull off their little beards and soak them in ice-cold water to get rid of any debris. Toss any mussels with cracked shells or any that don't open when cooked, and you're good to go!

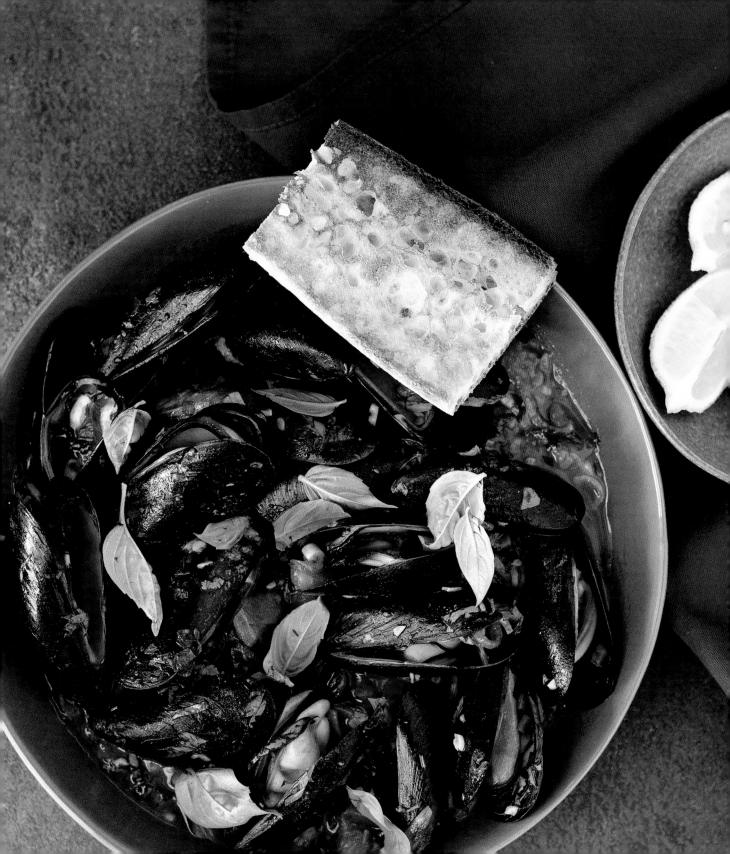

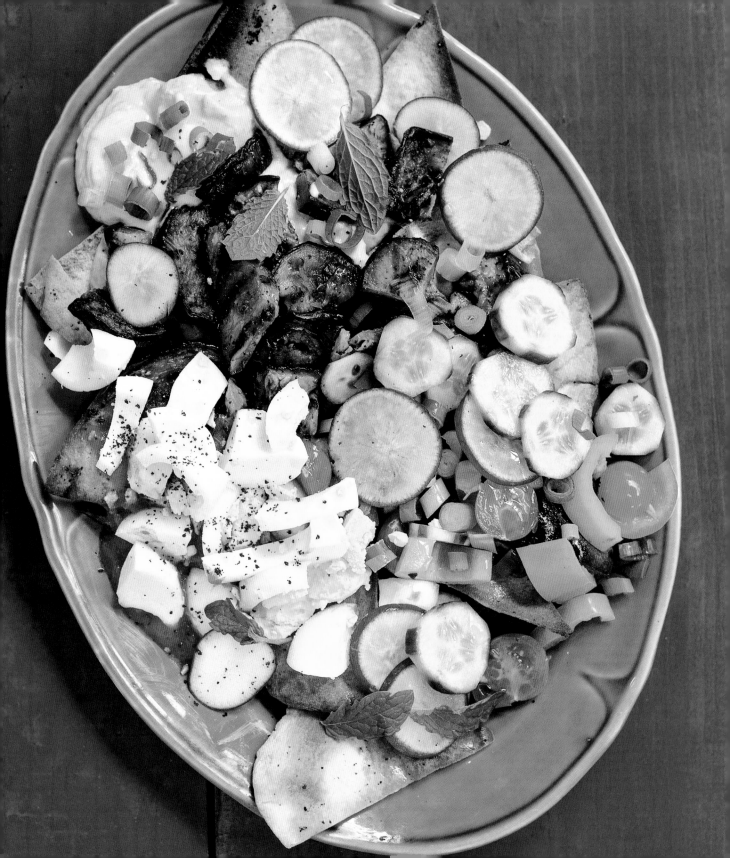

PITA NACHOS WITH FRIED EGGPLANT AND ALL THE TOPPINGS

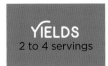

YIELDS
2 to 4 servings

These pita nachos are a fun play on the popular Israeli street food called sabich. Sabich is a stuffed pita pocket filled with fried eggplant, boiled eggs, spicy herb sauce, tahini and pickles, though variations do occur. Here, I took all those distinctive flavors and broke them up a bit into a fun and easy-to-throw-together appetizer. But I wouldn't judge you if this were your dinner, either.

Spiced Baked Pita Chips
(page 42)

½ tsp salt, divided

1 medium-sized eggplant, sliced into ½-inch (1.2-cm) thick slices

½ tsp ground sumac

½ tsp garlic powder

¼ cup (60 ml) olive oil, divided

1 small Persian cucumber, chopped into ½-inch (1.2-cm) pieces

1 small-medium tomato, seeded and chopped into ½-inch (1.2-cm) pieces

1 green onion, chopped finely

2 radishes, sliced thinly

Pepper

1–2 tbsp (15–30 ml) lemon juice

TOPPINGS
2 hard-boiled eggs, chopped

Harissa Sauce (page 144)

Hummus (page 159)

Tahini

Fresh mint leaves

Pickled jalapeños or Quick Pickled Vegetables (page 41)

Layer the pita chips on a platter and set aside.

Sprinkle ¼ teaspoon of salt over the eggplant and allow it to sit for 5 to 8 minutes. The salt will help pull out the moisture from the eggplant. Use a paper towel to blot off any excess moisture and season both sides of the eggplant evenly with sumac and garlic powder.

Heat a grill pan or outdoor grill on high and drizzle with 2 tablespoons (30 ml) of olive oil. Grill the eggplant slices on both sides until charred on the outside and softened inside, about 2 to 3 minutes total. Chop the eggplant into small pieces and set aside.

In a small bowl, toss together the cucumber, tomato, green onion and radish along with 2 tablespoons (30 ml) of olive oil, ¼ teaspoon of salt, pepper and a squeeze of lemon juice.

To layer the nachos, top the pita chips with the eggplant, eggs, chopped salad and dollops of harissa, hummus and tahini. Garnish with mint and pickles, if desired.

GRILLED ZA'ATAR-SPICED FLATBREAD
WITH SQUASH BLOSSOMS

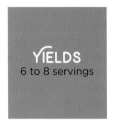

This is one of my favorite Mediterranean mezzes, and thanks to store-bought pizza dough, it's easy to whip up. Called man'oushe in Lebanese, this is quite similar to a flavored flatbread or pizza and is perfect as a snack or for breakfast. You can use any toppings you like with the za'atar, but if summer is at its peak, fresh squash flowers can't be beat. Other suggestions are baby spinach, thinly sliced zucchini ribbons, arugula and crumbled feta.

Serve alongside Magical Herb Tahini Sauce (page 147) or Cucumber, Yogurt and Mint Dip (page 160) for dipping.

1 lb (453 g) pizza dough, at room temperature

¼ cup (28 g) Homemade Za'atar (page 15)

¼ cup (30 ml) olive oil

6 squash blossoms, cut in half, or zucchini ribbons

Zest of 1 lemon

½ tsp salt

Magical Herb Tahini Sauce (page 147) or Cucumber, Yogurt and Mint Dip (page 160), for serving

Preheat an outdoor grill or a grill pan to high heat, or if using the oven, preheat to 475°F (246°C) and place a pizza stone in the oven to heat up while you prepare the recipe.

Divide the dough in half and roll out each piece to about 6 to 8 inches (15 to 20 cm) and set aside.

In a small bowl, whisk together the za'atar and olive oil and spoon the mixture over the two flatbreads, leaving a border around the edge.

Top the flatbreads with the squash blossoms and lemon zest and sprinkle ¼ teaspoon of salt on each one.

Cook the flatbreads until the edges slightly bubble and puff up and the dough is cooked through. Remove them to a wire rack and cool for a few minutes before cutting. Serve alongside tahini sauce or cucumber yogurt.

TIPS: There are several ways to cook the flatbread, and my two favorites are either on an outdoor grill or grill pan, or in the oven with a baking steel or baking stone. Either will provide a gorgeous crispy crust and chewy texture.

Squash blossoms are often found at farmers' markets when zucchini is at its peak. If blossoms are not in season, use a vegetable peeler to peel zucchini ribbons instead, which will provide a lovely freshness against the earthy za'atar spice.

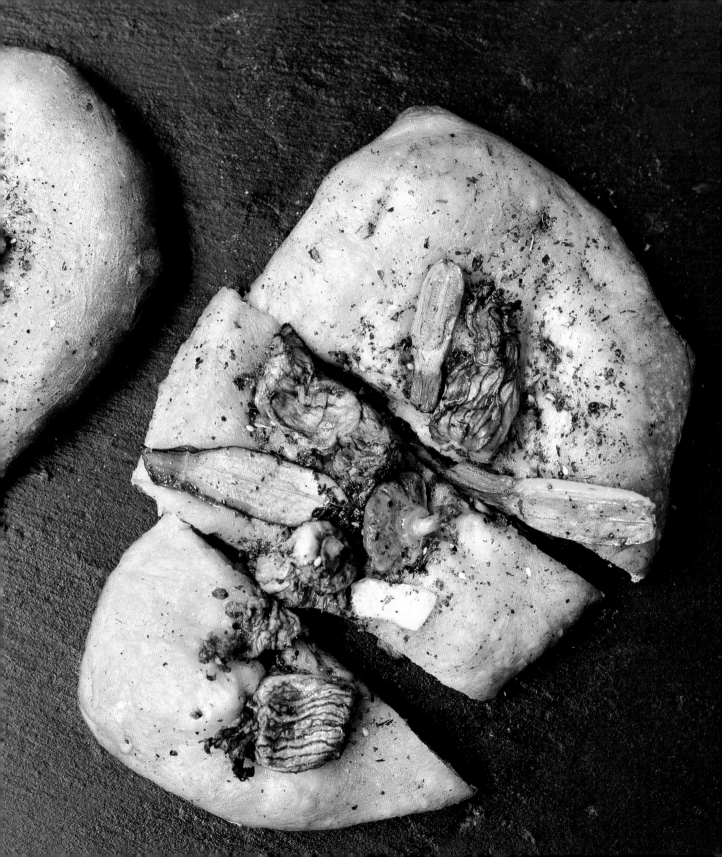

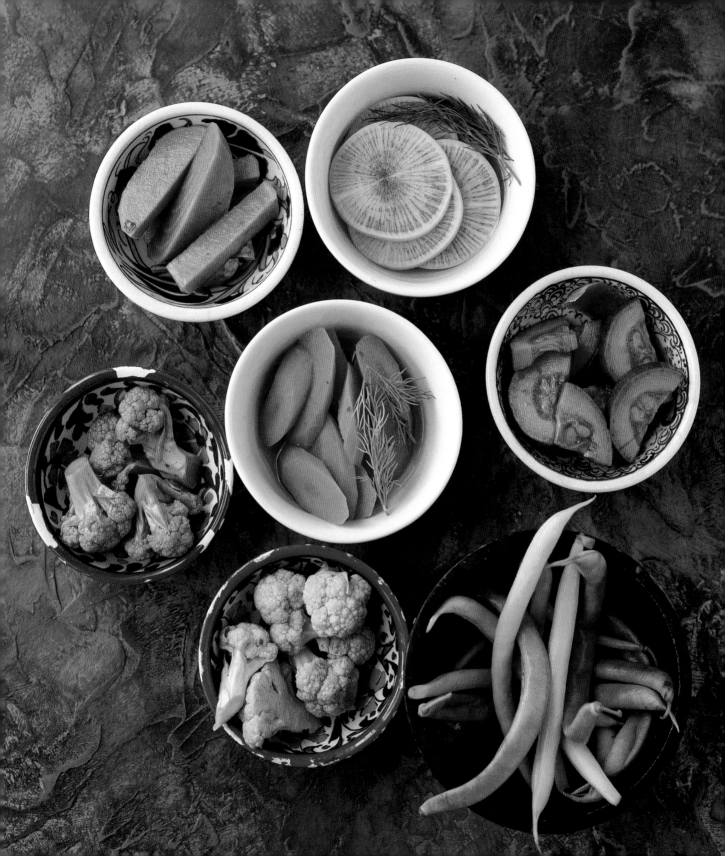

QUICK PICKLED VEGETABLES

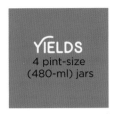

YIELDS
4 pint-size
(480-ml) jars

I will pickle anything if you give me the chance, and quick pickles are so easy to do with a simple pickling solution. Mediterraneans love their pickles and will pickle anything from lemons to peppers to the favorite rose-colored turnips to keep the season's memory. You'll often find pickles served on any mezze platter and alongside my favorite crispy falafel, which provides a lovely sharp bite to complement the savory taste. Serve quick pickles alongside Red Lentil Falafel (page 111), Za'atar Chicken Skewers (page 65) or as part of a mezze platter or snack.

VEGETABLES TO PICKLE

Persian or kirby cucumbers

Green beans

Cauliflower cut into small florets

Radish, sliced thin

Bell peppers, cut into small wedges

Onion or shallot, sliced thin

Carrots, diagonally sliced into ½-inch (1.2 cm) pieces

Roasted beets, also used to color vegetables pink

Chopped turnips

SPICES AND FLAVORINGS

1 inch (2.5 cm) peeled red beet, for color

2–3 whole garlic cloves per jar

Fresh mint, thyme, rosemary, sage or oregano

2–3 strips lemon or orange zest per jar

1 tsp Aleppo or red pepper flakes per jar

Slices of serrano or fresno pepper to taste

PICKLE SOLUTION

2 cups (475 ml) water

1 cup (240 ml) white vinegar

1 cup (240 ml) red wine vinegar

2 tbsp (36 g) salt

½ cup (96 g) white sugar

Clean four pint-size (480-ml) jars, making sure they are completely dry. Fill each jar with the desired vegetables and the beet, garlic, herbs, zest, Aleppo pepper and serrano pepper. Make sure to pack the jar with as many vegetables as you can, but leave about ¼ inch (6 mm) of headspace at the top of the jar. This will give the jar contents enough room for expansion.

In a small pot, combine the water, vinegars, salt and sugar and bring to a gentle boil, making sure all the sugar and salt is dissolved. Cook for 3 to 5 minutes and then pour the mixture into the jars. Be sure that all the vegetables and seasonings are submerged in the liquid.

Close the jars with lids and cool to room temperature. The pickles can be eaten as soon as the next day, but the longer they sit, the more flavorful they will be.

Store the pickles in the refrigerator for up to 1 month.

 TIP: The flavor options are endless, so have fun! Use different herbs and spices, in-season vegetables and different chilies for additional heat.

SPICED BAKED PITA CHIPS

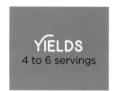

YIELDS
4 to 6 servings

Gone are the days of buying overpriced, unhealthy bagged pita chips, because they are so incredibly easy to make at home. Raid your spice drawer and toss with your favorite flavors, but I like to keep it classic and simple. A good toss with za'atar, garlic powder and olive oil is all you need. Add baked pita chips to your favorite salad for an extra crunch. Try them with Fennel Fattoush Salad with Pistachios (page 86), alongside Baked Feta Two Ways (page 22) or as a snack with Everyday Hummus (page 159).

4 pita breads, cut into 8–10 wedges

2–3 tbsp (30–45 ml) olive oil

½ tsp salt

2 tsp (6 g) za'atar

1 tsp garlic powder

½ tsp ground cumin

Finely chopped parsley leaves, for garnish

Preheat the oven to 400°F (204°C) and line a baking sheet with foil.

Toss the pita bread wedges with olive oil, salt, za'atar, garlic powder and cumin and arrange in a single layer on baking sheet.

Bake the pitas for 10 to 12 minutes until golden brown or a bit longer if you want them crispier. Garnish with chopped parsley.

Eat warm or allow to cool to room temperature before storing.

 TIP: Keep baked pita chips stored in either an airtight container or resealable plastic bag at room temperature and away from moisture for up to 4 days.

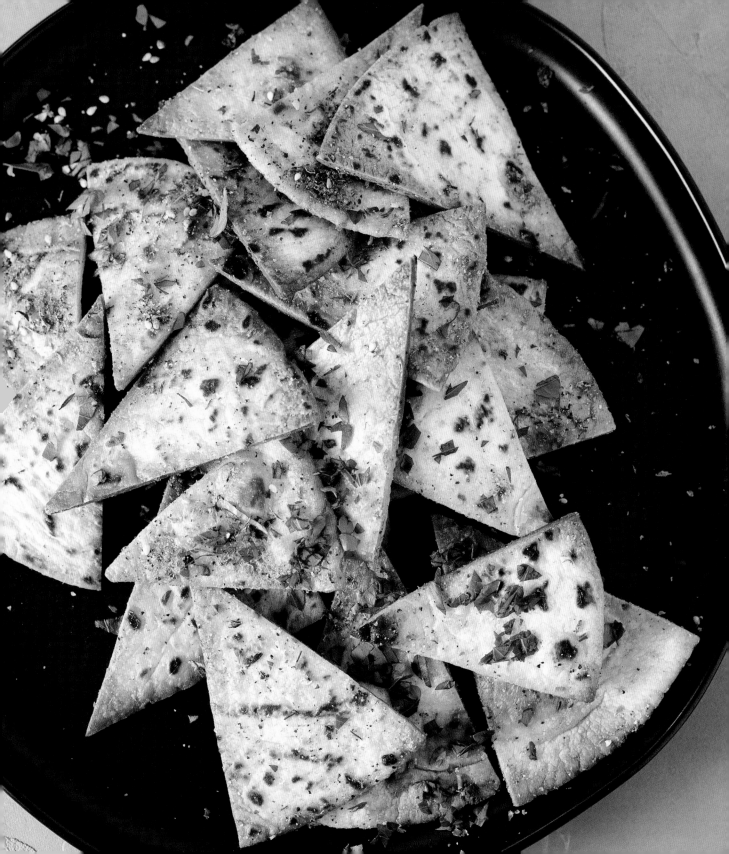

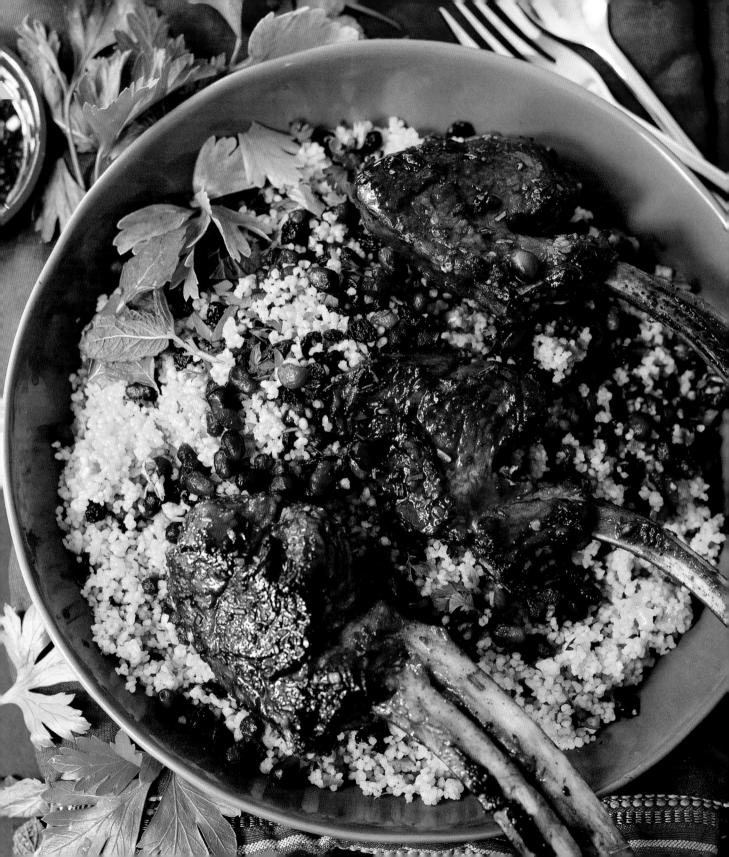

CHAPTER 2

THE MAIN MEAL

EASY AND VIBRANT MEDITERRANEAN DINNERS

My favorite time of the day is making dinner. It's a time to unwind and reflect on the day and let the creative juices flow with a glass of wine or a cocktail because let's be honest, it's a weeknight and we deserve one.

Truth be told, I am not a planner, especially when it comes to cooking. I have a tendency to change my mind a million times throughout the day and get instantly inspired by something I read or a new spice I discover. And after a busy day of the usual, I want something delicious but without hours of cooking time. That is why I can't emphasize enough on how important is it to keep a well-stocked pantry with healthy staples.

These Mediterranean meals are full of flavor without adding heaviness. Fresh produce, lean proteins and healthy cooking with olive oil create comforting meals without feeling overly heavy. Bold flavors of smoked paprika and bright sumac, for instance, transform a standard weeknight dinner into something exciting and nourishing.

One-Pot Paprika Chicken with Olives and Orzo (page 49) is a busy person's dream. The entire dish is done in one pot, and the flavors are exciting. Shakshuka with Lamb and Spices (page 46) is the perfect dinner and tastes like a gorgeous thick ragu—just make sure you have extra crusty bread to sop up all the delicious sauce. In the summer, turn on the grill and make Yogurt-Marinated Lamb and Eggplant Kabobs (page 54) or Za'atar Chicken Skewers (page 65), both done in under 20 minutes. And because we made it through the week, let's treat ourselves to an elegant night in with Pomegranate-Glazed Lamb Chops (page 61).

SHAKSHUKA WITH LAMB AND SPICES

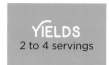
YIELDS
2 to 4 servings

If there were one reason I would eat an entire loaf of bread, it would be for this shakshuka. The ground lamb and spicy tomato sauce cook down together, creating the most luscious ragu. And then when you break into that yolk of the slowly poached eggs; it's all over. Yes, you'll need more bread to sop up all that delicious sauce. If you can't find ground lamb, ground beef would be just as delicious.

1 tsp olive oil

½ lb (226 g) ground lamb

1 shallot, chopped

1 red bell pepper, seeds removed and chopped into ¼-inch (6-mm) pieces

2 garlic cloves, chopped finely

1 fresno or serrano pepper, chopped and seeds removed (optional for less heat)

1 tsp tomato paste

1 tsp ground cumin

1 tsp paprika

1 tsp ground sumac, plus more for garnish

½ tsp Aleppo pepper flakes, plus more for garnish

½ tsp salt

1 (14.5-oz [411-g]) can whole plum tomatoes, with liquid

4 whole eggs

Chopped parsley, for garnish

Bring a 10-inch (25.4-cm) skillet or cast iron pan to medium-high heat. Add the olive oil and the lamb. Use a wooden spoon or spatula to help break up the meat and cook until thoroughly cooked through. If too much fat develops, carefully pour some out.

Add the shallot and bell pepper and continue cooking until they begin to soften, about 3 to 4 minutes.

Add the garlic and fresno pepper and cook for another minute so the garlic can soften and lightly caramelize.

Stir in the tomato paste, cumin, paprika, sumac, Aleppo pepper and salt. As you add in the tomatoes, use your hands to roughly break them up—be careful to not splatter tomato juice everywhere.

Stir everything together, making sure all the spices, lamb and tomatoes are blended well.

Use the back of a spoon to make 4 wells into the sauce. Crack 1 egg directly into each well, leaving the yolk exposed. Bring the temperature down to create a constant low simmer. Cook for another 5 to 7 minutes or until the eggs reach the desired doneness. You may want to cover the pan with a lid to help cook the tops of the eggs more evenly.

Garnish with parsley and an extra sprinkling of sumac and Aleppo pepper. Serve immediately with lots of crusty bread.

 TIP: Crack the eggs separately into a small bowl instead of directly into the pan, just in case you get a bad egg or bit of shell.

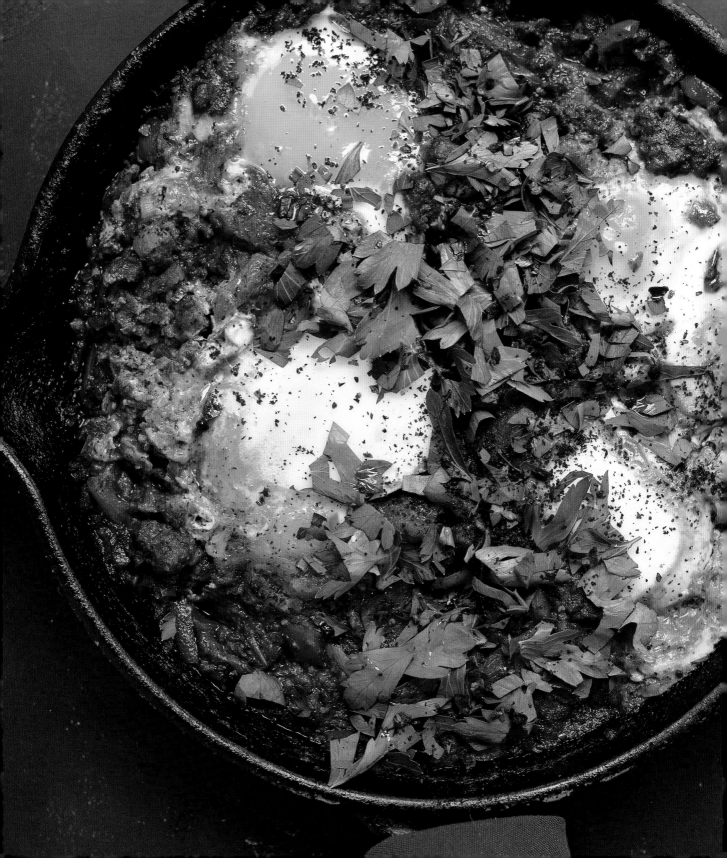

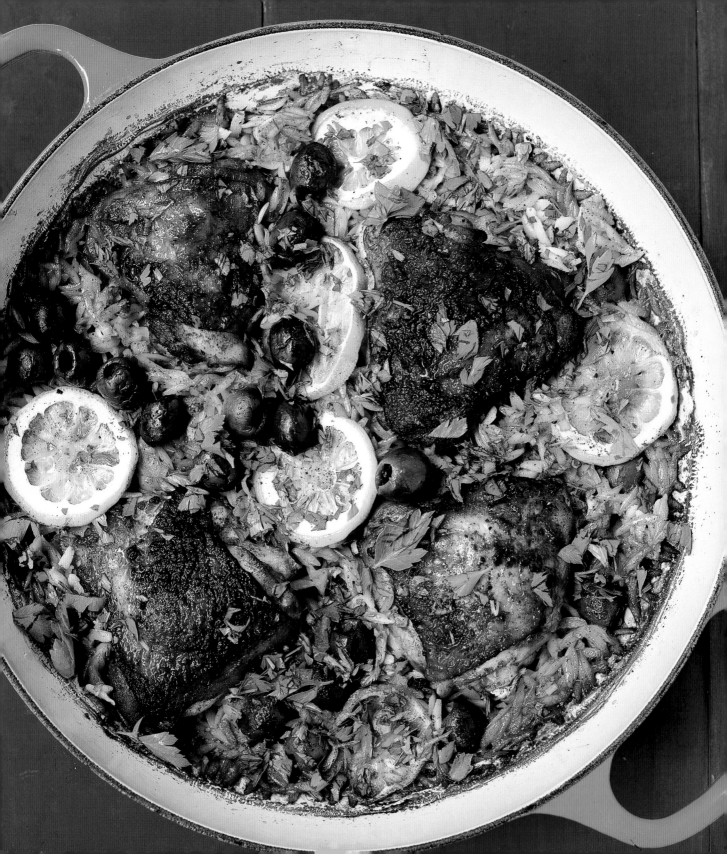

ONE-POT PAPRIKA CHICKEN
WITH OLIVES AND ORZO

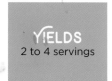

YIELDS
2 to 4 servings

This is a take on my mom's memorable paprika chicken. I have very fond memories of cleaning the whole bird and then rubbing it down with loads of paprika for weeknight dinners. The spice gives a deep rich color and imparts a delicious smoky flavor. This is my updated and modernized variation of mom's simple recipe made into an easy one-pan meal. Oh, and find yourself some Castelvetrano olives—they are buttery with a bit of brine and are oh-so-addictive.

2 lb (907 g) chicken thighs, bone-in and skin-on

2 tsp (5 g) smoked paprika

½ tsp salt

Olive oil, as needed

1 shallot, chopped finely

2 garlic cloves, chopped finely

8 oz (226 g) dried orzo

2 cups (475 ml) chicken stock

1 lemon, sliced

1 cup (150 g) whole pitted Castelvetrano olives

Chopped parsley, for garnish

Preheat the oven to 350°F (176°C).

In a bowl, toss the chicken with the paprika and salt, making sure the spices evenly coat the chicken.

Heat a large skillet over medium-high heat and add enough olive oil to coat the bottom. Don't add too much oil because the chicken will give off its own fat, as well.

Once the oil is hot, place the chicken thighs skin-side down into the hot pan and cook until a deep golden brown, about 3 to 4 minutes, and then flip the chicken over to the other side and cook for an additional 3 minutes.

Once both sides of the chicken are deep golden brown, remove to a plate and set aside.

In the same hot skillet, add the shallot and sauté until lightly golden, about 2 to 3 minutes. Add the garlic and sauté for another minute.

Add the orzo and stir so it is coated in the oil and aromatics (this will give it great flavor). Use a spatula to even out the orzo. Add the chicken back into the pan, skin-side up and pour in the stock.

Scatter the lemon slices and olives over the chicken and orzo and place in the oven, covered, for 25 minutes. Remove the cover and continue cooking for an additional 12 to 15 minutes.

Once cooked, remove from the oven and garnish with parsley.

 TIP: If you can't find the specified olives, substitute with the easier-to-find green manzanilla olives.

POACHED FISH WITH CHICKPEAS, TOMATOES AND HERBS

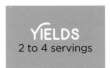

YIELDS
2 to 4 servings

This is such a delicious and versatile dish to prepare, and you don't need fancy fish-cooking skills, either. As the fish poaches in the aromatic broth, all the flavors infuse and create the most beautiful fragrant sauce that is perfect to spoon over the fish or your favorite side. Serve alongside Basmati Rice with Pistachios, Lima Beans and Dill (page 119) for a truly enjoyable meal.

2 tbsp (30 ml) olive oil

1 shallot, chopped

2 garlic cloves, chopped

1 tbsp (15 ml) tomato paste

8 oz (226 g) cherry tomatoes, cut in half

1 fresno or serrano pepper, thinly sliced, seeds removed for less heat

1 cup (164 g) cooked chickpeas

1 cup (240 ml) white wine

1½ cups (360 ml) water

1 lb (453 g) halibut, cut into 2 pieces

Salt, as needed

Freshly ground black pepper, as needed

1 lemon, zested and sliced thin

3–4 sprigs fresh oregano

3–4 sprigs fresh dill

Heat a large 13- to 15-inch (33- to 38-cm) skillet over medium heat and drizzle with olive oil. Add the shallot and sauté for 2 to 3 minutes until it softens but doesn't turn brown. Add the garlic and cook for another minute.

Add the tomato paste, cherry tomatoes, fresno pepper and chickpeas and toss together, making sure the tomato paste coats everything.

Pour in the wine and water and season the fish with salt and pepper. Nestle the fish into the broth so that it's submerged and top everything with lemon zest, lemon slices, oregano and dill.

Cover the skillet and bring the heat down to low-medium. Cook for 10 to 12 minutes until the fish is just cooked through. Depending on how thick the fish is, the cooking time may vary so check accordingly.

Once done, serve immediately and spoon the broth over the fish along with the tomatoes and chickpeas.

TIP: If halibut is not available, use any other mild fish, such as cod or tilapia, though the cooking time may be less since these fish cuts are usually thinner and will cook more quickly. The broth is also delicious with sea bass and salmon.

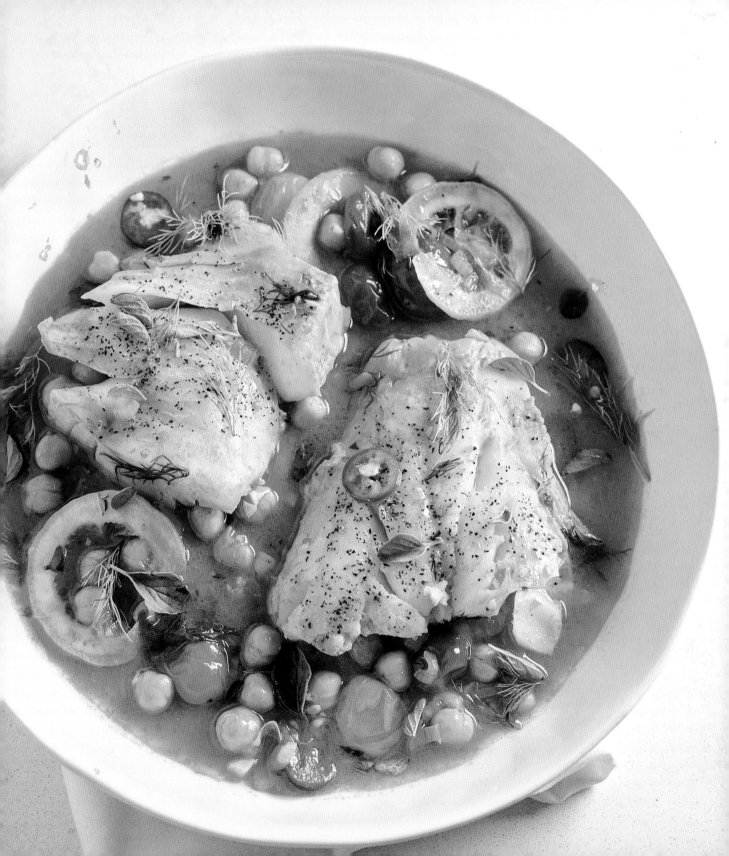

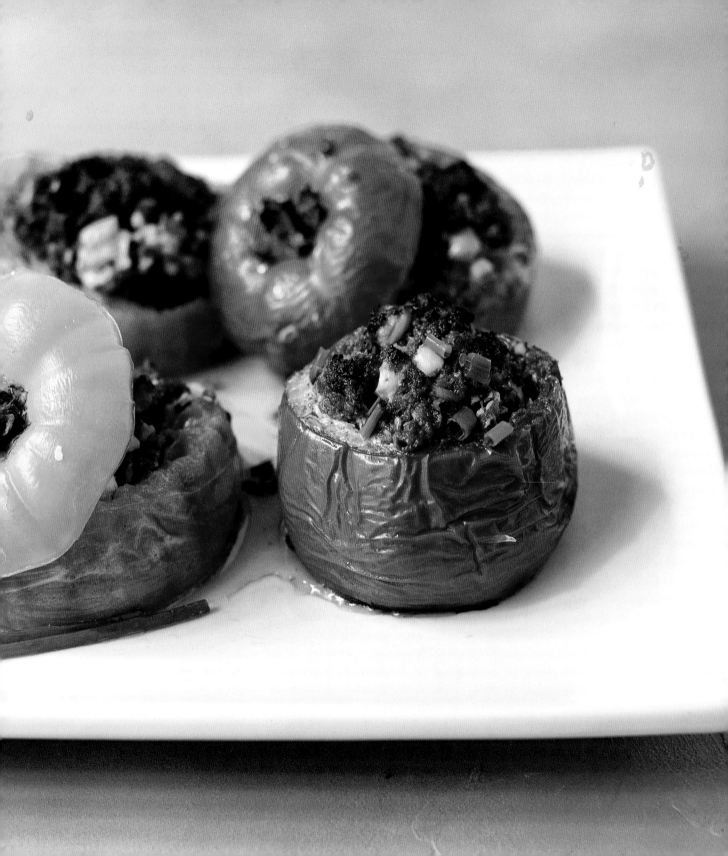

STUFFED TOMATOES WITH LAMB AND FETA

YIELDS
6 stuffed tomatoes

Late summer is when to make this recipe, and it will be worth the wait. The tomatoes slowly roast and impart their sweetness to the Mediterranean flavors of ground lamb, cumin, garlic and salty feta. Serve with Turmeric Lemon Couscous with Currants (page 112).

6 medium-sized tomatoes

1 lb (453 g) ground lamb

3 garlic cloves, chopped finely or grated

4–5 sprigs fresh oregano, stems removed and chopped

1½ tsp (4 g) paprika

1 tbsp (7 g) za'atar

1 tsp ground cumin

½ tsp Aleppo pepper flakes

Zest of 1 lemon

½ cup (75 g) crumbled feta cheese

½ tsp salt

2 tbsp (30 g) olive oil, plus more for garnish

Chopped chives, for garnish

Lemon wedges, for serving

Preheat the oven to 400°F (204°C) and line a baking sheet with foil. You can also use a rectangular baking dish.

Cut off the top third of the tomatoes, saving the lid and using a spoon to scoop out the flesh and any extra liquid from the tomatoes, leaving the tomato shells intact. Set aside.

In a medium-size bowl, add the ground lamb, garlic, oregano, paprika, za'atar, cumin, Alepo pepper, lemon zest, feta and salt. Mix everything together until well combined.

Stuff the tomatoes with the meat mixture and place on a baking sheet with the tomato lid on the side.

Drizzle the tomatoes with olive oil and bake for about 28 to 30 minutes. The tomatoes should be softened and slightly wrinkled and the meat mixture cooked through.

Garnish with fresh chives and serve with lemon wedges and top with the tomato lid if desired.

 TIP: The meat mixture itself is delicious in burger or meatball form, as well. Make a batch and freeze for easy use.

YOGURT-MARINATED LAMB AND EGGPLANT KABOBS

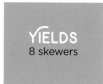

YIELDS
8 skewers

I love marinating proteins in yogurt. The acidity tenderizes the meat and leaves a gorgeous coating. The lemon zest and juice brings brightness, and when blended with smoky spices and fresh herbs, creates the most glorious marinade. Make an extra batch of the sauce and use it as a dip for the kabobs. Feel free to substitute another favorite vegetable, such as zucchini, for the eggplant. If lamb isn't available, substitute beef cubes or chicken breasts. The marinade is versatile enough to use on any of your favorite proteins.

½ cup (120 ml) olive oil

½ cup (120 ml) plain 2% or full-fat Greek yogurt

3 garlic cloves, chopped

1 lemon, zested and juiced

½ tsp ground cumin

½ tsp ground turmeric

½ tsp salt

½ tsp Aleppo pepper flakes

¼ cup (5 g) packed mint, stems removed

¼ cup (5 g) packed parsley, hard stems removed

¼ cup (5 g) packed cilantro, hard stems removed

1 lb (453 g) leg of lamb, cut into 1-inch (2.5-cm) cubes

1 large eggplant, cut into 1-inch (2.5-cm) cubes

Charred lemon halves, for serving

If using wooden skewers, soak for at least 30 minutes so they don't burn. If using metal skewers, skip this step.

Preheat a charcoal or gas grill on medium-high.

Using a food processor or blender, pulse together the oil, yogurt, garlic, lemon zest and juice, cumin, turmeric, salt, Aleppo pepper, mint, parsley and cilantro until everything is incorporated and the marinade is smooth. Taste for seasoning and reserve about half of the marinade for dipping.

Use paper towels to pat dry the cubed lamb. This will help the marinade stick to the meat better. Add both the cubed lamb and the eggplant to a large bowl or resealable plastic bag.

Pour the rest of the yogurt mixture over the lamb and eggplant and mix to evenly coat. Slide 4 to 5 lamb cubes onto each skewer and about 4 to 5 eggplant cubes each onto separate skewers. You will use 8 skewers altogether.

Place the skewers on the grill and cook on all sides, until desired doneness, about 10 to 12 minutes.

Serve with the reserved yogurt sauce for dipping and a squeeze of charred lemon.

 TIP: If you have the time, marinate for at least 30 minutes to overnight, which will only make the meat more tender and flavorful.

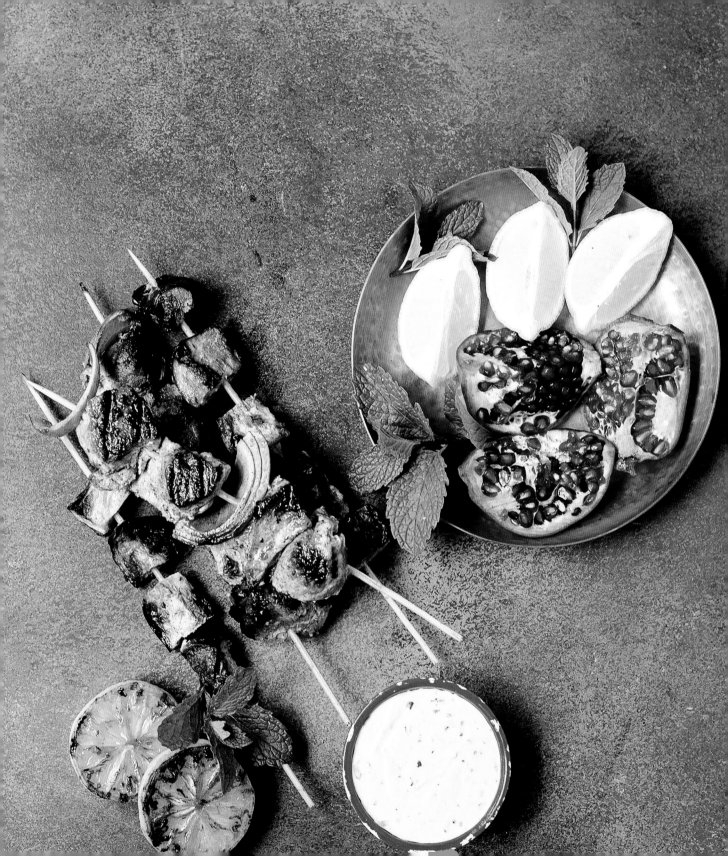

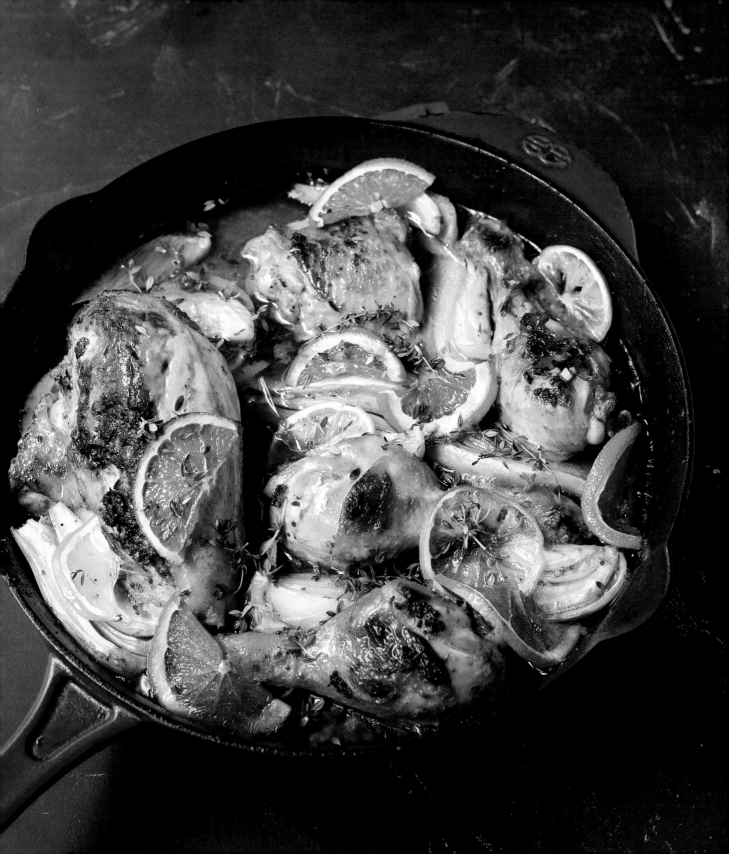

OLIVE OIL-BRAISED CHICKEN
WITH FENNEL AND CITRUS

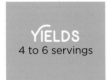

YIELDS
4 to 6 servings

This dish is everything I love about Mediterranean cooking and is one of my favorite recipes from my blog. Simple, bright, fresh ingredients create the most beautiful and healthy dinner. Citrus and fennel work perfectly together and infuse the braised chicken with flavor. Mustard, the secret ingredient, ties it all together. Serve with Cucumber, Yogurt and Mint Dip (page 160) on the side or Basmati Rice with Pistachios, Lima Beans and Dill (page 119).

1 bone-in and skin-on chicken breast (about 8–10 oz [226–283 g])

3–4 skin-on chicken drumsticks

2 garlic cloves, chopped finely

2 tbsp (30 ml) stone ground mustard

½ lemon, zested and juiced

½ orange, zested and juiced

1 tsp ground turmeric

4–5 sprigs fresh thyme, leaves removed, plus more for garnish

½ tsp salt

Freshly ground pepper

1 cup (240 ml) olive oil

1 fennel bulb, fronds and stems removed and cut into eighths

½ lemon, sliced thin

½ orange, sliced thin

1½ cups (360 ml) chicken stock, plus more if needed

Preheat the oven to 425°F (218°C).

Pat dry the chicken pieces with a paper towel and place in a large bowl. Add the garlic, mustard, lemon and orange zest and juice, turmeric, thyme, salt and pepper. Massage the marinade all over the chicken and marinate for at least 20 minutes.

Heat a large 13- to 15-inch (33- to 38-cm) cast iron skillet over medium heat and pour in the olive oil. Carefully place the chicken in the pan and sear on each side so the outside is a deep golden color, about 3 minutes per side.

Once the chicken is seared, add the sliced fennel, lemon and orange slices and more thyme sprigs. Pour in the chicken stock and bring to a gentle simmer for about 2 to 3 minutes.

Carefully place the skillet in the oven and cook for about 25 minutes, or until the chicken is fully cooked. As the chicken cooks, use a ladle to spoon braising liquid over the chicken midway through cooking.

Once the chicken is done, the sauce should be thickened and the fennel and citrus charred and tender. Allow the chicken to rest for 5 minutes before serving.

STUFFED EGGPLANT WITH MEAT AND TAHINI

YIELDS
4 servings

It wouldn't be a Mediterranean cookbook without some sort of stuffed eggplant. Here, I used some of my favorite Turkish flavors such as smoky cumin and spicy Aleppo pepper and smooth nutty tahini for some flavor and texture contrast. Top with Blood Orange and Pomegranate Salsa (page 164) for an added kick.

2 medium-large eggplants, cut in half lengthwise

2 tbsp (30 ml) olive oil, plus more for drizzling

1 lb (453 g) ground beef

1 small white onion, chopped finely

2 garlic cloves, chopped finely

1 medium-sized tomato, seeded and chopped

1 tbsp (15 ml) tomato paste

1 tsp ground cumin

1 tsp Aleppo pepper flakes

½ tsp paprika

½ tsp salt

½ cup (120 ml) tahini

Blood Orange and Pomegranate Salsa (optional, page 164), for serving

Finely chopped cilantro leaves, for garnish

Preheat the oven to 425°F (218°C).

Using a small paring knife cut out the eggplant flesh, leaving a ½-inch (1.2-cm) border around the inside of the eggplant. This will help hold the filling. Chop up the removed eggplant flesh and set aside.

Drizzle a large skillet with the olive oil over medium heat. Add the ground beef and cook until mostly cooked through. Make a space in the center of the pan and add the onions. Cook together until the onions are softened, another 3 to 4 minutes.

Add the chopped eggplant and garlic and cook everything together until the eggplant softens and the garlic is cooked. Use a large spoon to help break up the eggplant and meat so it becomes one homogenous mixture.

Add the tomatoes, tomato paste, cumin, Aleppo pepper, paprika and salt and stir everything together. Taste for seasoning.

Arrange the eggplant shells on a foil-lined baking sheet, stuff the meat mixture inside the eggplant and drizzle the tops with olive oil. Bake for 18 to 20 minutes until the eggplants are cooked and deepened in color.

Serve with tahini and top with pomegranate salsa and cilantro, if desired.

TIP: When picking out an eggplant, look for the smaller, younger ones that are far less bitter and less seedy. Also make sure the eggplant has a nice smooth outer skin with no visible dents or bruising.

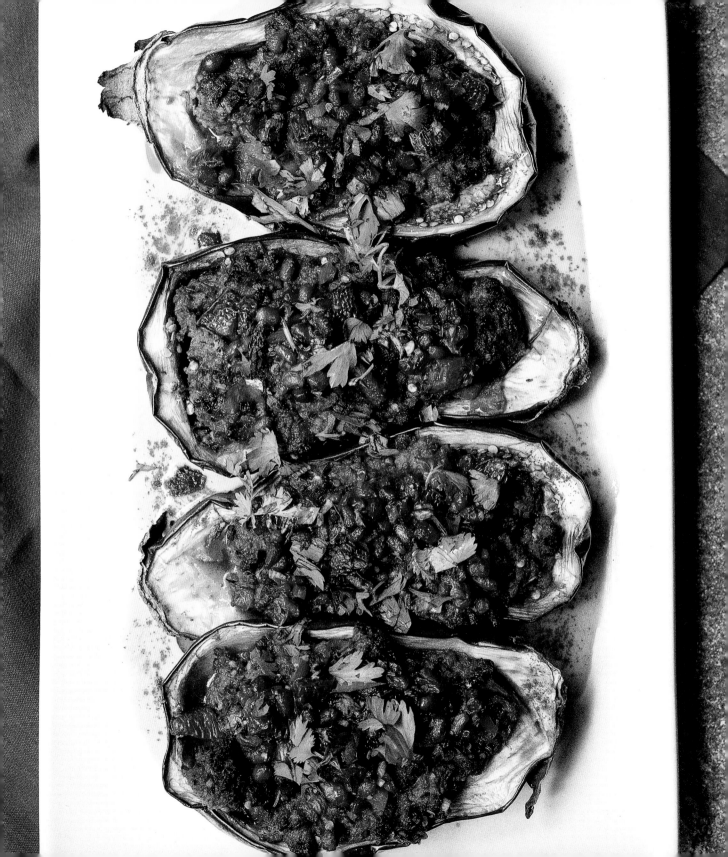

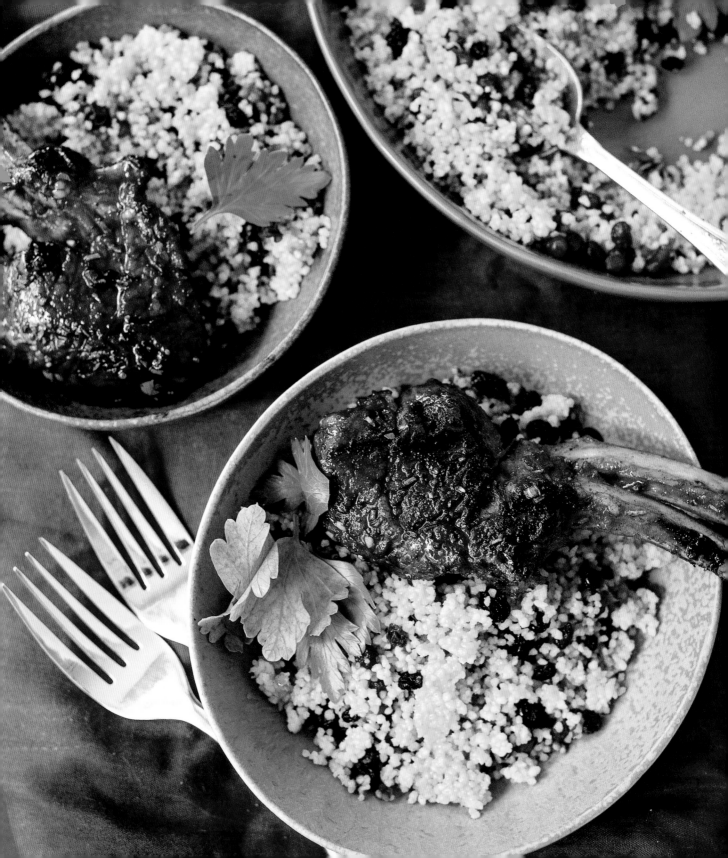

POMEGRANATE-GLAZED LAMB CHOPS

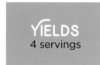

YIELDS
4 servings

This dish is the ultimate showstopper, not only for looks, but for flavor as well. The marinade base is pomegranate molasses, a thick syrupy sauce made from reduced pomegranate juice with sugar and lemon. It's potent and tangy and glazes over the grilled meat beautifully. Serve the lamb chops alongside Turmeric Lemon Couscous with Currants (page 112) and Easy Homemade Harissa Sauce (page 144) for added heat.

2 lb (907 g) rack of lamb, cut into individual chops (about 8–10 chops)

¼ cup (60 ml) pomegranate molasses

¼ cup (60 ml) olive oil

1 clove garlic, chopped finely

1 small shallot, chopped finely

4 sprigs rosemary, leaves removed and chopped

½ tsp ground cinnamon

½ tsp ground cloves

1 tsp ground sumac

½ tsp Aleppo pepper flakes

½ tsp salt

Use a paper towel to pat dry the lamb chops on all sides, which will help the marinade stick to the meat.

In a large resealable plastic bag, pour in the molasses, oil, garlic, shallot, rosemary, cinnamon, clove, sumac, Aleppo pepper and salt and mix everything together. Pour out ¼ cup (60 ml) of the mixture and reserve for later use. Place the lamb chops in the bag and coat thoroughly with the marinade. Allow the lamb to marinate for at least 20 minutes but no more than 1 hour.

Heat a grill pan (or charcoal/gas grill) to high heat and cook the lamb chops on each side for 2 to 3 minutes for medium-rare or until the desired doneness.

Remove to a platter and brush the reserved marinade all over the meat.

 TIP: Pomegranate molasses is becoming easier to find in grocery stores so be sure to check in your local store's international aisle.

EVERYDAY CHICKEN SHAWARMA

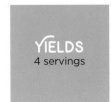

YIELDS
4 servings

Everyone should have a go-to shawarma recipe that doesn't require having an upright spit in your kitchen. A loose interpretation of the *New York Times* version, my everyday shawarma is quick and easy to prepare and is one of those dishes where you dump the entire spice drawer into the recipe to infuse the meat with a deep savory flavor. Pair this with the Magical Herb Tahini Sauce (page 147) and wrap it up in some crisp lettuce leaves or flatbread. This is also delicious shredded over Chopped Rainbow Salad with Crispy Lavash (page 98) or Fennel Fattoush Salad with Pistachios (page 86).

2 lb (907 g) boneless, skinless chicken thighs

¼ cup (60 ml) olive oil

5 garlic cloves, chopped finely

2 lemons, zested and juiced

1½ tsp (4 g) ground sumac

½ tsp Aleppo pepper flakes

½ tsp ground allspice

2 tsp (5 g) ground cumin

2 tsp (5 g) paprika

1 tsp ground turmeric

¼ tsp ground cinnamon

1 tsp kosher salt

TO SERVE

Pita bread

Magical Herb Tahini Sauce (page 147)

Chopped salad

Fresh herbs

Lemon wedges

Preheat the oven to 400°F (204°C).

In a large bowl, combine the chicken thighs with the oil, garlic, lemon zest and juice, sumac, Aleppo pepper, allspice, cumin, paprika, turmeric, cinnamon and salt and coat everything well. Cover with plastic wrap and marinate in the fridge for at least 20 minutes and up to an hour, the longer the better.

Transfer the chicken to a foil-lined baking sheet. Pour the marinade over the chicken. Bake for 30 to 35 minutes until the chicken is cooked through. For extra crispy edges, increase the heat to 425°F (218°C) and continue cooking for 8 to 10 minutes.

Remove the chicken from the oven and allow it to rest for 5 minutes before cutting into it; then cut the chicken into slices.

Serve with pita bread, tahini sauce, chopped salad, fresh herbs and lemon.

 TIP: If you'd like to substitute chicken breasts for thighs, use a rolling pin to pound the chicken to an even thickness. This will tenderize the chicken and help it to be just as moist as the chicken thighs.

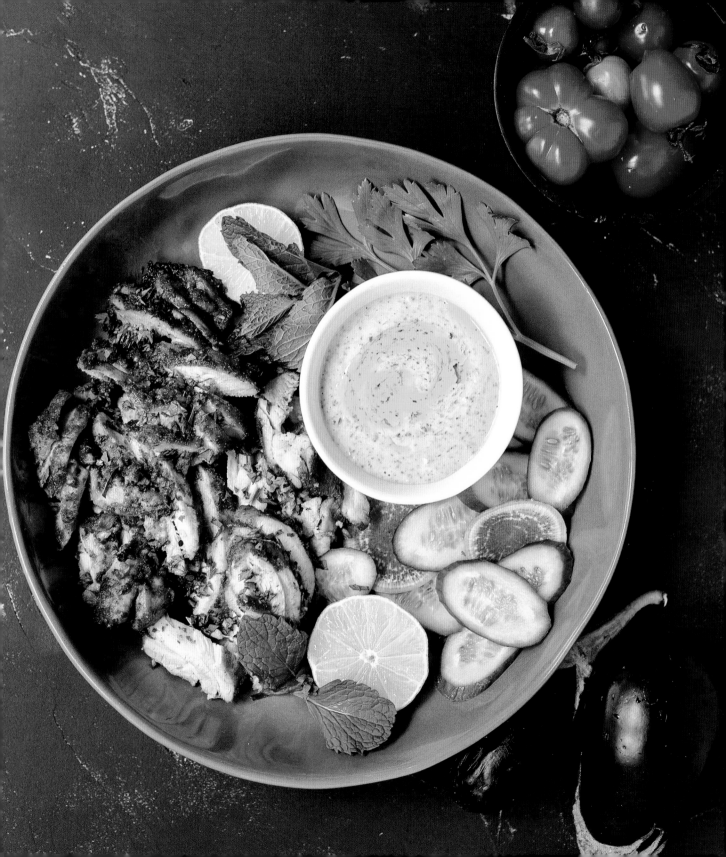

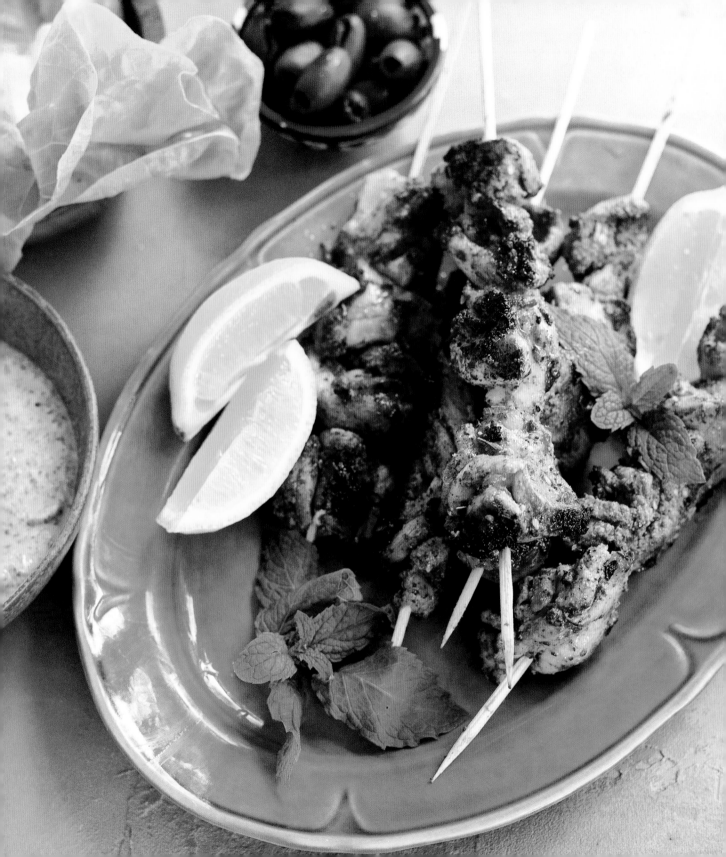

ZA'ATAR CHICKEN SKEWERS

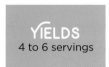

YIELDS
4 to 6 servings

I love a simple and powerful spice rub. If you have the time, marinate the chicken for as long as you can so the flavors can develop. Serve with pita bread or, for an even healthier option, serve with fresh crisp lettuce leaves along with spicy Easy Homemade Harissa Sauce (page 144) or Magical Herb Tahini Sauce (page 147) and Quick Pickled Vegetables (page 41).

2 lb (907 g) chicken thighs, cut into 1-inch (2.5-cm) pieces

1 tbsp (15 ml) olive oil

2 tbsp (14 g) za'atar

1 tsp allspice

½ tsp salt

½ tsp Aleppo pepper flakes

TO SERVE

Pita bread

Lettuce leaves

Magical Herb Tahini Sauce (page 147)

Quick Pickled Vegetables (page 41)

If using wooden skewers, soak for at least 30 minutes so they don't burn when grilled.

In a large bowl or resealable bag, add the chicken, oil, za'atar, allspice, salt and Aleppo pepper and massage everything together well. Marinate the chicken for at least 20 minutes.

Preheat a charcoal or gas grill or grill pan on high heat and skewer 4 to 5 pieces of chicken onto each skewer.

Grill the chicken on both sides until fully cooked, about 10 to 12 minutes total.

Once done, remove from the grill and allow to rest for a few minutes. Serve alongside pita bread, lettuce leaves, tahini sauce and pickles.

SLOW-COOKER BEEF STEW WITH GREEN BEANS, POTATOES AND SPICES

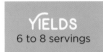
We call this simple and rustic stew fasulye in Turkish. I often make a large batch in the slow cooker. If I start it in the morning, by dinnertime the entire house smells wonderful. My addition of cinnamon and paprika brings out an exotic warmness and makes the stew taste even better the next day.

2 lb (907 g) beef chuck, cut into 1-inch (2.5-cm) cubes

1 tsp paprika

½ tsp ground cinnamon

½ tsp ground cumin

½ tsp Aleppo pepper or other red pepper flakes

½ tsp salt

1 lb (453 g) Yukon potatoes, quartered

3–4 garlic cloves, chopped

1 small white onion, sliced thin

1 (15-oz [425-g]) can white beans, drained

3 cups (710 ml) tomato sauce

3 cups (710 ml) water

1 cup (150 g) green beans (fresh or frozen)

Freshly chopped parsley, for garnish

Lemon wedges, for garnish

Cooked rice, for serving

Lay out the cubed beef and use a paper towel to pat the cubes dry on both sides. This will help the spices stick and not slide right off. Add the cubed meat to a bowl and toss with paprika, cinnamon, cumin, Aleppo pepper and salt so everything is coated evenly.

Add the seasoned meat to the slow cooker and top with the potatoes, garlic, onion, white beans, tomato sauce and water.

Use a spatula to gently stir everything together. Scatter the green beans on top and close the lid. Cook on low for 6 to 7 hours or on high for 3 to 4 hours. The meat should be tender enough to tear with a fork. Taste for seasoning and garnish with parsley. Serve with lemon wedges and cooked rice.

 TIP: Add the green beans on top of everything so the beans "steam" rather than overcook in the stew. Serve fasulye with cooked white rice for a hearty and delicious dinner that feeds a crowd.

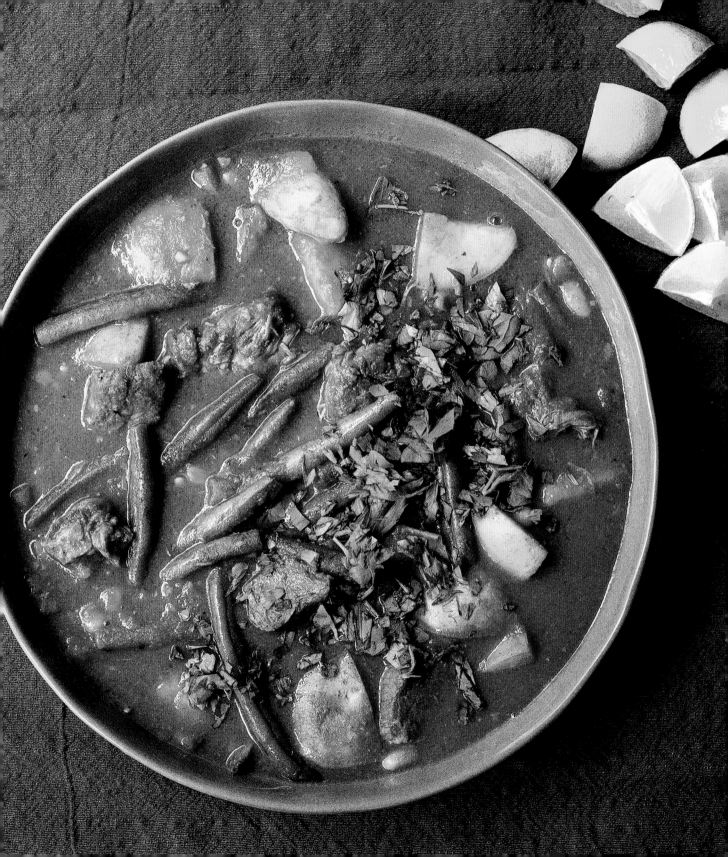

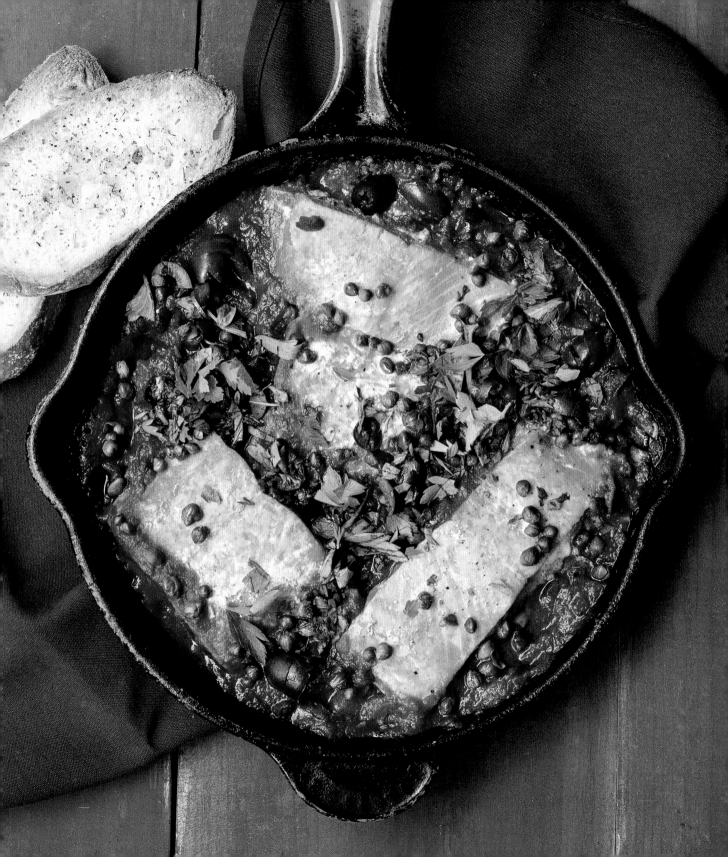

SALMON PUTTANESCA

If I could live off any flavor profile for the rest of my life, it would be salty, garlicky and briny. Puttanesca has always been a favorite because it's flavor packed and quickly prepared. The secret ingredient is the anchovy fillets that melt into the simmering olive oil to perfume the entire dish. Serve with a side of rice, pasta or just a big hunk of toasted garlic bread to sop up all of the delicious sauce.

2 tbsp (30 ml) olive oil

4 anchovy fillets

3 garlic cloves, chopped finely

½ white onion, chopped finely

¼ cup (60 ml) red wine

1 cup (240 ml) tomato sauce

1 lb (453g) salmon fillets, bones and skin removed, cut into 4-oz (113-g) portions

¼ tsp salt

Black pepper, as needed

3 tbsp (25 g) capers

¾ cup (100 g) Kalamata olives, pitted and roughly chopped

Fresh parsley, as needed for garnish

Toasted garlic bread, for serving

Drizzle enough olive oil in a 10-inch (25-cm) skillet to almost coat the bottom of the pan and bring to medium heat. Add the anchovies and use a spatula to break them up in the olive oil until you can't see any more pieces.

Add the garlic and sauté for another minute. Add the onions, sautéing until they turn a light golden color, about 3 to 4 minutes.

Add the red wine to deglaze and reduce for a minute so the wine thickens. Add the tomato sauce and gently stir everything together.

Season both sides of the salmon with salt and pepper and nestle the fillets into the sauce and scatter capers and olives all around. Lower the heat to a gentle simmer and cover the skillet with a lid, poaching the salmon in the sauce until cooked, about 5 to 7 minutes.

Once done, garnish with parsley and serve with toasted garlic bread.

 TIP: The term "deglazing" refers to using a liquid (wine in this case) to disolve browned bits from the bottom of the pan. It intensifies the dish's flavor and is a good base for any sauce.

SAFFRON SHRIMP WITH TOMATOES AND FETA

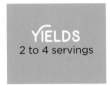

YIELDS
2 to 4 servings

My best friend and I used to enjoy a dish very similar to this when we were teenagers growing up in Hawaii. We would have girls' night out at a local seafood spot overlooking the ocean. We would order a strawberry lemonade and a very memorable shrimp-feta-tomato dish served with pasta. It's been 15 years since we ate there, but we still talk about this dish. This homage to our teenage years is updated with the twist of white wine and saffron. Serve with Persian Rice with Turmeric and Saffron (page 123).

¼ tsp loosely packed saffron

2 tbsp (30 ml) warm water

3 tbsp (45 ml) olive oil

1 large shallot, chopped

3 garlic cloves, thinly sliced

¼ cup (60 ml) white wine

1 lb (453 g) medium-sized shrimp, peeled and deveined

½ tsp salt

½ tsp Aleppo pepper flakes

1 medium tomato, chopped

4 oz (113 g) feta cheese, roughly crumbled

Basil leaves, for garnish

Lemon wedges, for garnish

In a small bowl, steep the saffron in the warm water for a few minutes.

In a large skillet over medium-high heat, drizzle in the olive oil. Add the shallot and sauté for 2 to 3 minutes until it turns a light golden brown and softens.

Add the saffron and water and stir into the oil. Add in the garlic and continue sautéing until the garlic is a light golden color, for another 1 to 2 minutes. Add the wine and reduce for 1 to 2 minutes.

Add in the shrimp and season with salt and Aleppo pepper, stirring everything together. Add in the tomato and continue cooking until the shrimp is opaque and the tomatoes have released their juices and softened.

Taste for seasoning and remove from the heat. Add in the feta and garnish with basil leaves and lemon wedges.

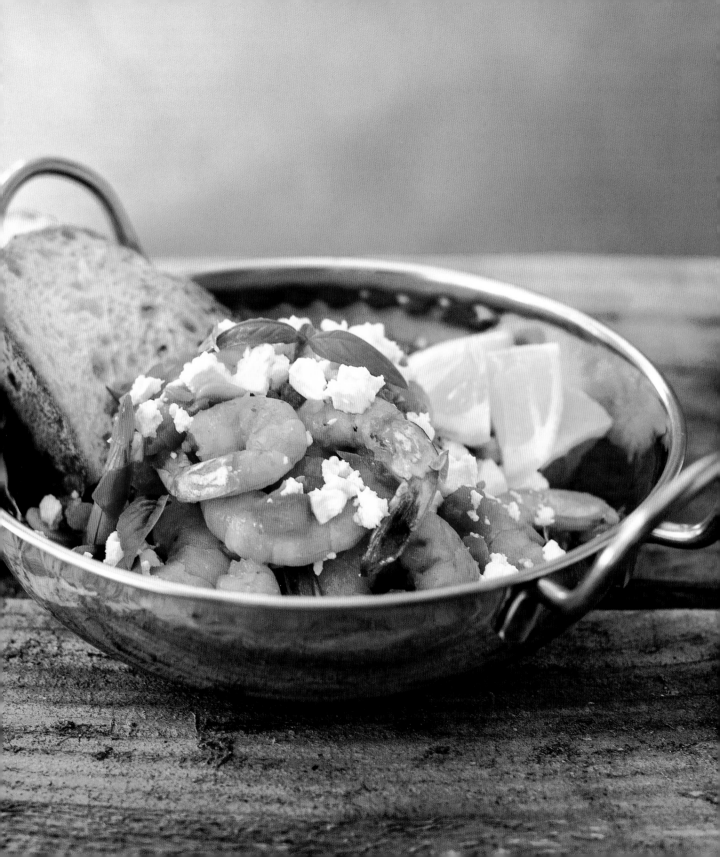

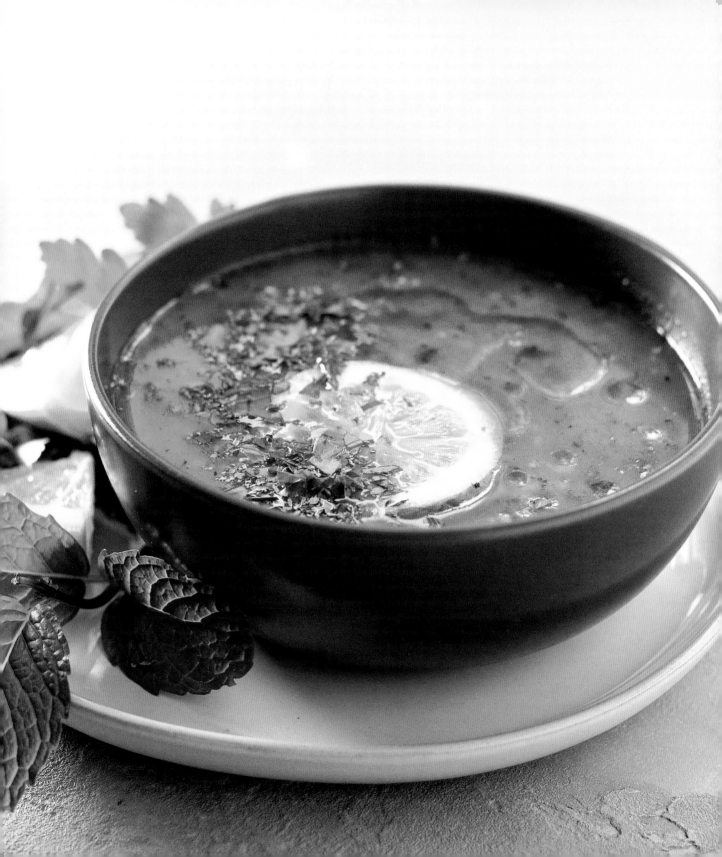

CHAPTER 3

SOUPS AND SALADS

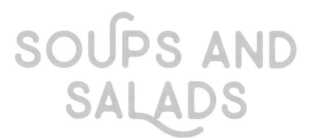

FLAVORFUL ONE-POT MEALS

It took a while to convince my husband, Joe, that a soup or salad still qualifies as a meal. And I get it—I need to feel satisfied as well. That's why I promote my mottos of "no more wimpy salads" and "no more wimpy all-I-taste-is-water soups."

Enjoying a salad should mean enjoying a big beautiful bowl filled with crunch, texture and different flavor profiles. I love adding fruit to my salads for a touch of sweetness, like in the Sweet-and-Spicy Chopped Salad (page 89) or Jeweled Tabbouleh Salad with Couscous (page 97) with citrus and pomegranate seeds. Have fun with seasonal ingredients. On a cool fall day the Autumn Squash Salad with Figs and Arugula (page 101) will surely warm and fill you up in no time.

The soups in this chapter are full of my favorite seasonings. Robust flavors of cinnamon with tomatoes and smoky paprika-infused oil permeate the dishes. And the best part, all of the soups in this chapter are quick and easy and done in mostly under 40 minutes on the stove. One pot, simple ingredients, 40 minutes and you have enough to feed a whole family plus more for your freezer.

Turkish Lentil Soup (page 77) is one of my most popular recipes from the blog, and the first recipe I made after we traveled to Turkey. It is full of healthy grains, smoky paprika and bright lemon juice to round it all out. And for those tomato soup lovers, Roasted Pepper and Tomato Soup with Broiled Halloumi Cheese (page 74) is dreamy, especially topped with that broiled halloumi cheese. This one is for those rainy days where you want a little spice to cozy up to.

I love making extra batches of soups and stocking them in the freezer. I pour extra soup, about two to four servings, into a freezer strength resealable bag, lay it flat to freeze and just pile them up. Then when I'm craving a bowl of comforting soup, I just pull one out and done.

ROASTED PEPPER AND TOMATO SOUP WITH BROILED HALLOUMI CHEESE

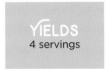
YIELDS
4 servings

I don't think I could write a cookbook and not have a recipe dedicated to my love of tomato soup. I took inspiration from my favorite condiment, harissa, and used the flavors to make a smooth and savory tomato soup. The best part? Sitting atop the soup is broiled halloumi cheese, which chars ever so gently, yet is still sturdy enough to handle the high heat.

3 whole red bell peppers

3 tbsp (45 ml) olive oil, plus more for garnish

1 medium leek, chopped, about 1 cup (125 g)

1 fresno or serrano pepper, chopped (seeds removed if you want less heat)

3 carrots, peeled and chopped into ½-inch (1.2-cm) pieces

2 garlic cloves, chopped

½ tsp ground cinnamon

1 tsp ground sumac

1½ tsp (2 g) dried oregano

½ tsp Aleppo pepper flakes

½ tsp salt, or to taste

1 (14.5-oz [411-g]) can diced tomatoes, with liquid

2–2½ cups (475–590 ml) vegetable or chicken stock

4 oz (113 g) cubed halloumi cheese

Lemon wedges, for garnish

Oregano leaves, for garnish

Preheat the oven to 400°F (204°C) and place the bell peppers on a foil-lined baking sheet. Roast the peppers for 20 to 25 minutes, turning mid-way through until they are charred on all sides and softened.

Remove the peppers from the oven and cover with another layer of foil for about 10 minutes. This will continue steaming the peppers and make it easier to remove the charred outer skin. Peel away any charred skin, so only the soft roasted pepper is left. Core and stem the peppers, roughly chop and put aside.

In a medium pot over medium high heat, add the oil, leek, fresno pepper and carrots and sauté for 3 to 4 minutes, until the leeks and carrots begin to soften.

Add the garlic, cinnamon, sumac, oregano, Aleppo pepper and salt and continue cooking for another minute until everything blends together.

Add in the tomatoes with liquid, roasted peppers and stock. Bring to a gentle boil. Cover and cook the soup for about 30 minutes.

Once done, blend the soup using an immersion blender until smooth. Taste for seasoning and add more stock if the soup is too thick. At this point, turn on the broiler.

Ladle the soup into 4 oven-safe bowls and top with about 1 ounce (28 g) of cheese. For easier transfer, place the soup bowls on a baking sheet and broil in the pre-heated oven until the cheese is lightly charred, about 2 to 3 minutes.

Remove from the oven and allow to cool for a few minutes. Garnish with squeeze of lemon juice, fresh oregano leaves and a drizzle of olive oil.

 TIP: To make things go a little quicker, use a 12-ounce (355-g) jar of roasted peppers in lieu of roasting them yourself.

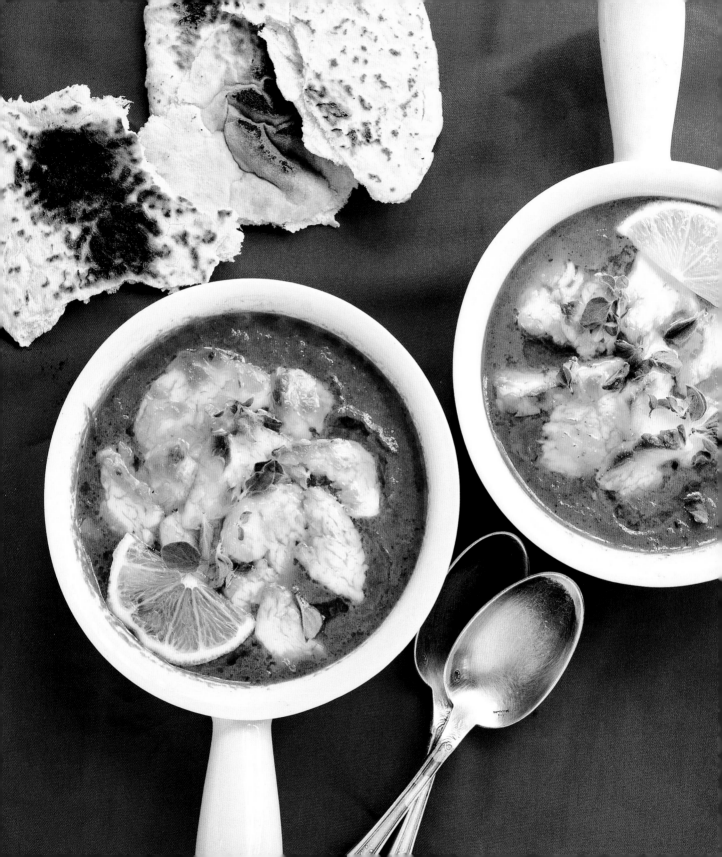

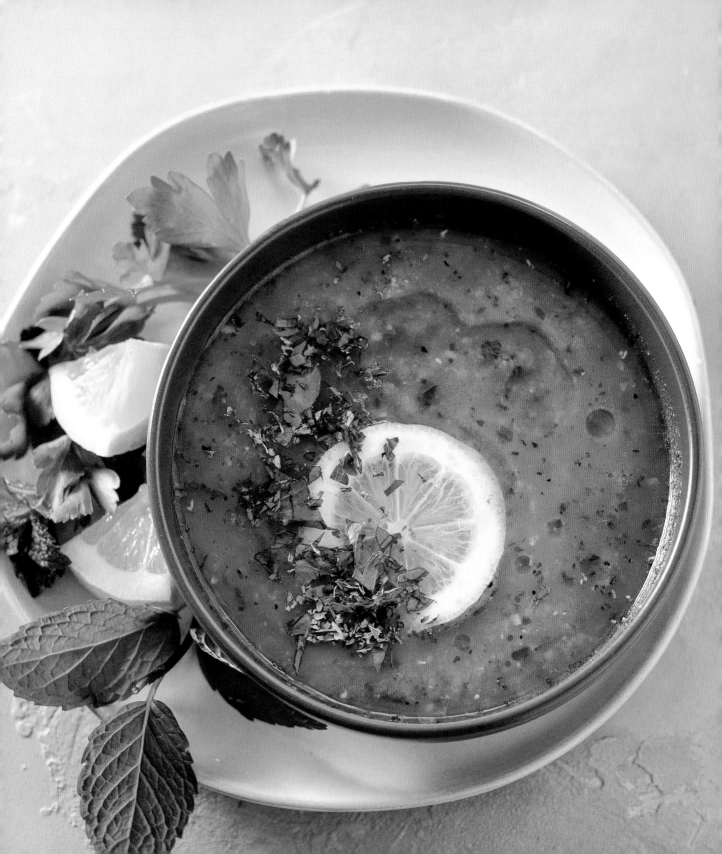

TURKISH LENTIL SOUP

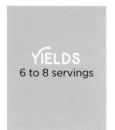

YIELDS
6 to 8 servings

This Turkish lentil soup is one of the most popular recipes on my blog and one of my favorites, as well. Inspired by one of the recipes in my favorite Turkish cookbook, *The Sultan's Kitchen*, this lentil soup has such fascinating layers of flavors with smoked paprika, tomato paste, fresh mint and lemon juice to brighten it all up.

When we were in Istanbul a few years ago, we enjoyed a bowl of very similar lentil soup in a tucked-away spot a few stairs below a busy bazaar. If you blinked, you would have walked right past it. The atmosphere was very modest, but eating that soup at that very moment is something I will never forget.

2 tbsp (30 g) butter

2 tbsp (30 ml) olive oil, plus more for garnish

½ red onion chopped finely, about 1 cup (160 g)

1 medium red bell pepper chopped, about 2 cups (300 g)

2 garlic cloves, chopped finely

1 tbsp (6 g) dried mint

1 tbsp (7 g) smoked paprika

½ tsp Aleppo pepper flakes

2 tbsp (30 ml) tomato paste

1 medium-sized tomato, seeded and chopped into 1-inch (2.5-cm) pieces

1 lemon, zested then cut into wedges for garnish

½ tsp salt, or more to taste

1 cup (192 g) dried red lentils

¼ cup (50 g) long grain Basmati rice

¼ cup (42 g) red or white quinoa

7–8 cups (1.6–1.9 L) vegetable or chicken stock

Parsley leaves, chopped, for garnish

Mint leaves, for garnish

In a large pot on medium heat, add the butter and oil and sauté the onion and pepper until tender, about 5 to 7 minutes.

Add the garlic and sauté until lightly caramelized, about 2 to 3 minutes. Add the mint, paprika and Aleppo pepper and stir everything together in the oil.

Stir in the tomato paste, tomato and lemon zest and season with salt and cook for another 1 to 2 minutes to soften the tomato.

Add the lentils, rice and quinoa and stir well. Pour in the stock and bring the soup to a low boil.

Cover the pot and cook the soup for about 30 to 35 minutes, until the rice and quinoa are tender. Taste for doneness and seasoning.

Once the soup is cooked, use an immersion blender to puree some of the soup for better texture or ladle a few cups into a blender or food processor and then add that back into the soup.

Serve the soup with a garnish of lemon wedges, olive oil, parsley and mint.

LEMONY CHICKEN SOUP WITH RICE

YIELDS
4 to 6 servings

Often known by its popular Greek name avgolemono, this soup is a very similar Turkish version that I grew up with. Done in nearly 30 minutes, this is a hearty, thick soup that feeds the whole family on a cool evening. Make it even easier with leftover roasted chicken and whisked-in egg yolks for added richness.

6 cups (1.4 L) chicken stock or broth

½ cup (92 g) basmati or jasmine rice, rinsed

2 cups (280 g) cooked, shredded chicken

2 egg yolks

4 tbsp (60 ml) lemon juice

1 tsp salt, or to taste

Pepper, to taste

Fresh parsley and mint, for garnish

Lemon slices, for garnish

In a large soup pot, bring the chicken stock to a boil and add in the rice. Reduce to a simmer and cover the pot, cooking until the rice is about halfway cooked, about 15 minutes.

Add in the shredded chicken and continue cooking until the rice is fully cooked, another 10 minutes.

In another bowl, whisk together the egg yolks and lemon juice and slowly stream in a ladle of the hot broth, whisking at the same time. This is called tempering and slowly brings the egg yolks up to the same temperature as the soup, so they don't cook too fast and curdle.

Turn off the heat and stir the egg mixture into the soup. Do not bring to a boil, or you may risk curdling the eggs.

Season with salt and pepper and garnish with parsley, mint, lemon slices and extra lemon juice.

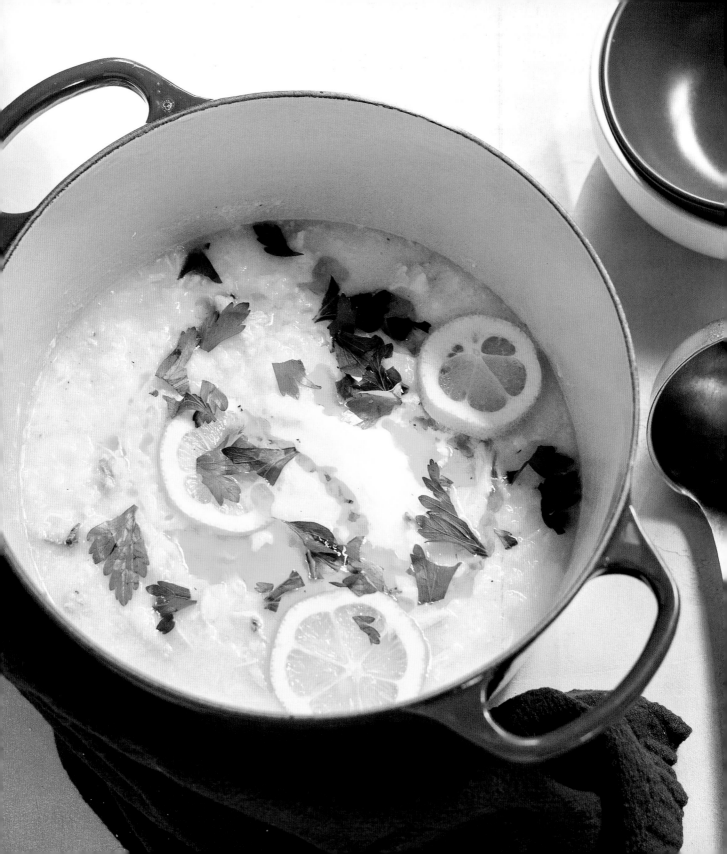

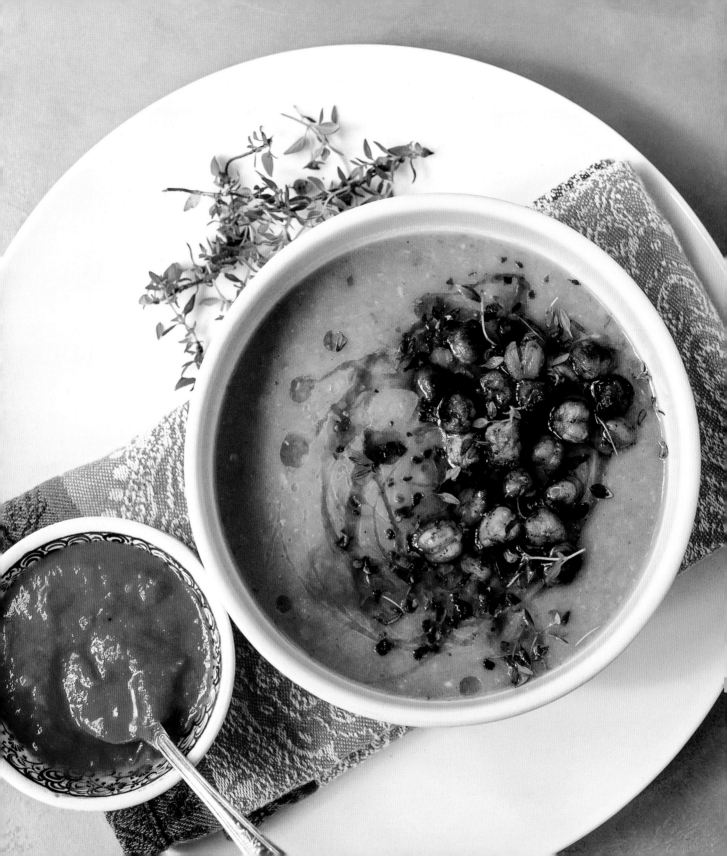

CUMIN-SCENTED SQUASH AND LENTIL SOUP WITH CRISPY CHICKPEAS

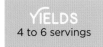
YIELDS
4 to 6 servings

A delicious soup does not need to take hours over the stove. Red lentils cook quickly, and if you roast the squash ahead of time, everything can be bowled up in under an hour. My favorite tool, the immersion blender, is used here, and it makes creamy soups a breeze. I highly recommend investing in one for your cooking essentials.

2 lbs (907 g) acorn or butternut squash or mixture of both, peeled and cut into 1-inch (2.5-cm) cubes

2 tbsp (30 ml) olive oil, divided

1 cup (164 g) cooked chickpeas

½ tsp ground cumin

½ tsp paprika

¼ tsp salt

SOUP

2 tbsp (30 ml) olive oil, plus more for garnish

1 small red onion, diced

1 fresno pepper, seeded and diced

1 tsp ground turmeric

1 tsp ground cumin

½ tsp paprika

½ tsp salt or more to taste

5 cups (1.2 L) vegetable or chicken stock, plus more if needed for consistency

1 cup (192 g) dried red lentils

Easy Homemade Harissa (page 144), for garnish (optional)

Fresh thyme leaves, for garnish

Preheat the oven to 400°F (204°C) and arrange the squash on a baking sheet. Drizzle with 1 tablespoon (15 ml) of olive oil and roast until fork tender, for about 1 hour.

While the squash cooks, make the roasted chickpeas on another baking sheet. Spread the chickpeas on a foil-lined baking sheet and dry thoroughly with a paper towel. Toss with cumin, paprika, salt and the remaining 1 tablespoon (15 ml) of oil and bake for 15 to 18 minutes. Once done, they should be crispy with a deep brown color. Remove from the oven and set aside until the soup is ready.

In a medium-size pot, coat the bottom with 2 tablespoons (30 ml) of olive oil and bring up to medium heat. Add the onion and fresno pepper and sauté until softened, about 3 to 4 minutes.

Add the turmeric, cumin, paprika and salt and stir thoroughly. Add the cooked squash, vegetable stock and lentils and gently stir everything together, making sure everything is submerged in the liquid. Add a bit more stock if needed.

Cover with a lid and bring the soup up to a gentle boil and cook until the lentils are tender, about 30 minutes.

Once done, turn off the heat and use an immersion blender to blend the soup to the desired consistency.

Ladle the soup into bowls and garnish with a drizzle of olive oil, harissa, crispy chickpeas and fresh thyme.

TIP: This soup freezes incredibly well. Make a large batch and pour into resealable bags for quick meals. Add crispy chickpeas just before serving.

WHITE BEAN SOUP 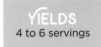 HERBS, LEMON AND ARUGULA

YIELDS
4 to 6 servings

There is nothing like a good bean soup that tastes like it was cooked for hours, yet the only work you did was raid your pantry. Thanks to canned chickpeas and white beans, this herby white bean soup is a breeze to make, not to mention hearty and healthy as well. If you don't have arugula on hand, substitute baby spinach leaves instead.

3 tbsp (45 ml) olive oil

2 ribs celery, diced

1 medium sized leek chopped, about 2 cups (320 g)

1 medium sized red or orange bell pepper chopped, about 2 cups (300 g)

1 carrot, peeled and sliced thin into ¼-inch (6-mm) pieces

3 garlic cloves, chopped

1 tbsp (3 g) dried oregano

2 sprigs rosemary, leaves removed and chopped

2 sprigs fresh oregano, leaves removed and chopped

2–3 sprigs fresh thyme, leaves removed and chopped

5 cups (1.2 L) vegetable or chicken stock

1 bay leaf

4 strips lemon zest, using a vegetable peeler

1-inch (2.5-cm) chunk Parmesan rind

15 oz (425 g) canned or cooked chickpeas, rinsed

15 oz (425 g) canned or cooked white beans, rinsed

¾ tsp salt, or to taste

½ tsp ground pepper, or to taste

2 cups (40 g) arugula, loosely packed

Parmesan strips, using a vegetable peeler, for garnish

Place a medium-size soup pot over medium heat and drizzle with olive oil. Add the celery, leek, bell pepper and carrot and sauté so they all begin to soften, about 5 to 6 minutes. Allow the vegetables to sweat but not turn brown—you just want them to soften.

Add the garlic, dried oregano, rosemary, oregano and thyme and continue to cook, stirring everything together for another minute. Pour in the stock and add the bay leaf, lemon zest, Parmesan rind, chickpeas and beans. Stir everything together and season to taste.

Cover the pot with a lid and bring to a low simmer and cook for 30 minutes.

Once done, remove the cheese rind and the lemon zest. If you prefer a creamier soup, use an immersion blender to blend some of the soup. Or ladle 2 cups (475 ml) into a blender or food processor and blend to a smooth consistency and then add that back in with the soup.

Turn off the heat and add the arugula. The residual heat will soften the leaves.

Garnish with strips of Parmesan.

 TIP: Save those Parmesan rinds! As soon as you're done with most of the cheese, store the rinds in a resealable plastic bag and keep them in the freezer. Use them to flavor soups, sauces and broths.

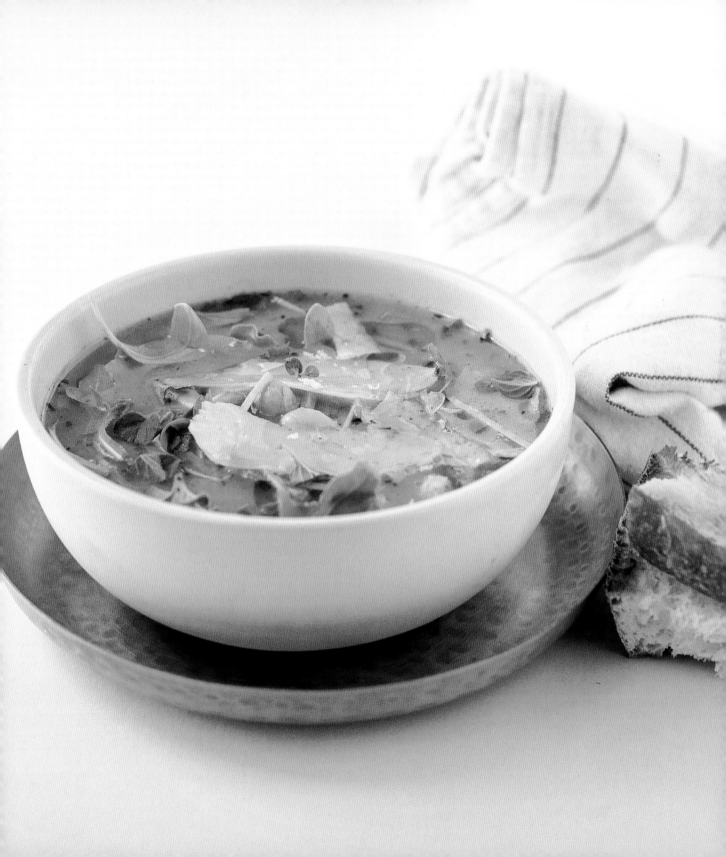

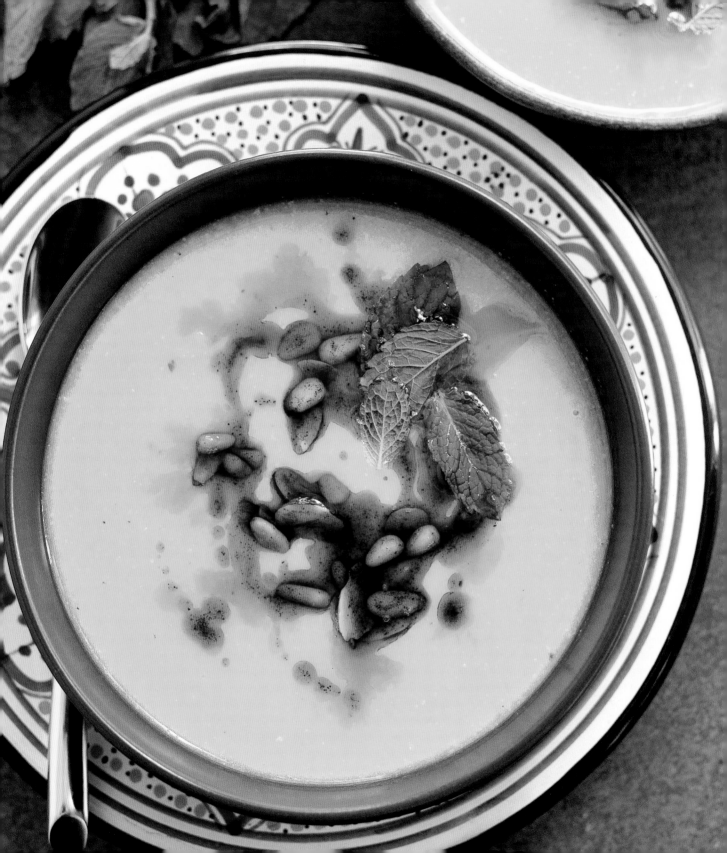

CREAMY SAFFRON CAULIFLOWER SOUP WITH PAPRIKA OIL

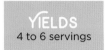

YIELDS
4 to 6 servings

It's a wonderful thing when you're served a bowl of silky smooth soup and later find out that there is absolutely no cream in the dish whatsoever. The addition of starchy potatoes helps smooth out the soup, giving it a luxurious feel. Garnish with smoky pine nuts and bright mint to round out the deep flavors.

3 tbsp (45 ml) olive oil

1 shallot, diced

4 garlic cloves, chopped

2 medium Yukon gold potatoes, unpeeled and cut into 1-inch (2.5-cm) pieces, about 2 cups (300 g)

1½–2 lb (680–907 g) white cauliflower, florets cut into 1-inch (2.5-cm) pieces

5 cups (1.2 L) vegetable or chicken stock

¾ tsp loosely packed saffron, roughly ground

½ tsp salt, or to taste

Ground pepper, to taste

PAPRIKA OIL WITH PINE NUTS AND ALMONDS

¼ cup (60 ml) olive oil

1 tsp smoked paprika

2 tbsp (12 g) sliced almonds

2 tbsp (17 g) pine nuts

Fresh mint leaves, for garnish

Place a medium-sized soup pot over medium heat and drizzle with the olive oil. Add the shallot and sauté until softened but not browned, about 3 to 4 minutes. Add the garlic and continue cooking for another 1 to 2 minutes.

Add the potatoes and cauliflower and pour in the stock. The vegetables should be submerged in the liquid, but if some are slightly poking out, that's OK, as they will cook down. Add in the ground saffron and season with salt and pepper and bring to a boil.

Cover with a lid and reduce the heat to medium low and cook until the vegetables are very tender, about 22 to 25 minutes. The vegetables should easily break when a fork or knife is inserted.

While the soup cooks, make the paprika oil with pine nuts. In a small sauté pan on medium heat, add the oil, paprika, almonds and pine nuts. Sauté until the almonds and pine nuts become fragrant and lightly toasted, about 2 to 3 minutes. Keep a close eye on it as this happens fairly quickly, and keep stirring so the nuts don't burn. When done, pour the nuts and oil into a small bowl.

Once the vegetables are done, use an immersion blender to blend the soup to a creamy mixture. You can also ladle the soup into a blender or food processor.

Ladle the soup into bowls and use a spoon to drizzle the paprika oil and nuts over the soup and garnish with fresh mint.

TIP: You can use all almonds or all pine nuts if you have one or the other on hand.

FENNEL FATTOUSH SALAD
WITH PISTACHIOS

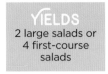

YIELDS
2 large salads or
4 first-course
salads

I've been working on the term, "no more wimpy salads" since I started my blogging career. There is far too much delicious produce in the world to make it limp and boring. Fattoush salad is a common Mediterranean salad full of crunchy vegetables and crispy pita chips. Usually fried, these pita chips are baked until crisp instead to serve their crunchy purpose.

PITA CHIPS

2 pita breads, cut into 8–10 wedges

Olive oil, as needed

1 tsp za'atar

½ tsp kosher or sea salt

CITRUS VINAIGRETTE

⅓ cup (80 ml) olive oil

1 tbsp (15 ml) honey

½ lemon, zested and juiced

1 tsp ground sumac

¼ tsp salt

Ground pepper

SALAD

1 large fennel bulb, peeled and sliced very thin using a mandoline, about 2 cups (300 g)

3 cups (75 g) baby arugula

¼ cup (40 g) chopped pistachios

½ cup (15 g) fresh mint leaves

Preheat the oven to 400°F (204°C). On a baking sheet covered in parchment paper, lay out the pita wedges and drizzle with the oil, za'atar and salt. Toss well so everything is evenly coated.

Bake the pita chips for 10 to 12 minutes or until golden brown and crisp. Once done, remove from the oven and set aside.

In a small bowl or glass jar, add the oil, honey, lemon zest and juice, sumac, salt and pepper and mix until combined to make the vinaigrette.

Assemble the fennel, arugula, pistachios, mint and pita chips in a large bowl. Add 3 tablespoons (45 ml) of the vinaigrette and toss together. The salad will be lightly coated with the dressing but not overly dressed. Taste for seasoning and add more vinaigrette as needed.

TIP: Unless you have exceptional knife skills, invest in a mandoline to shave the fennel into paper-thin slices. The thin fennel blends beautifully with the peppery arugula and it will all be the same size.

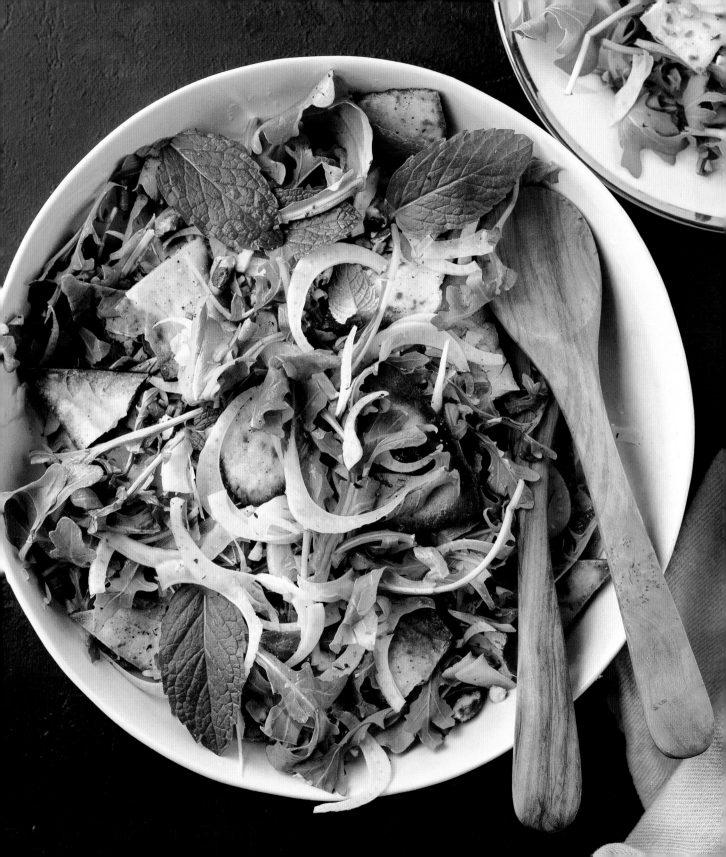

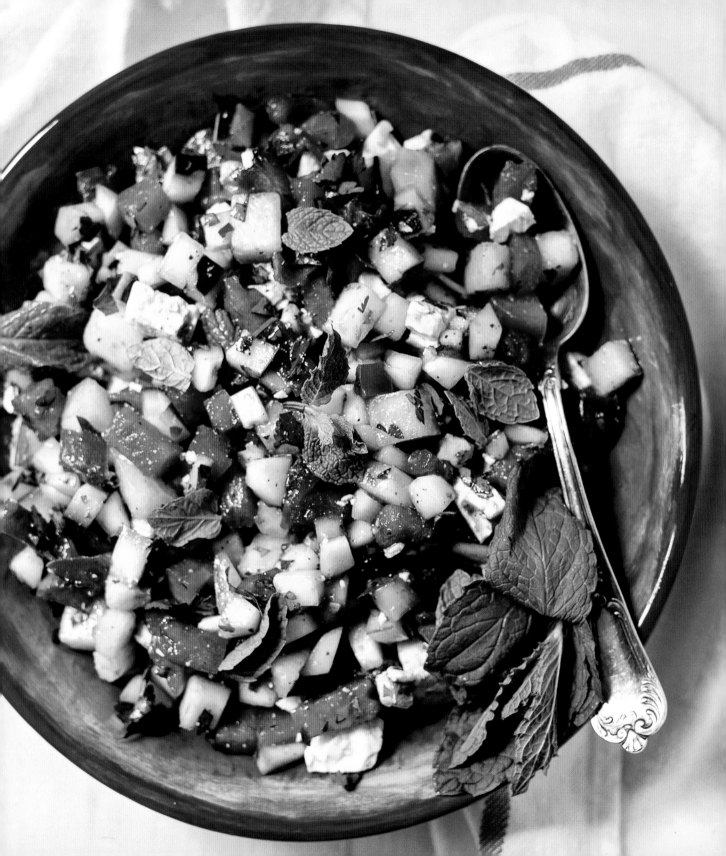

SWEET-AND-SPICY CHOPPED SALAD

YIELDS
4 servings
as a side

Traditional Israeli chopped salad does not have melon or chilies in it, but I love the sweet and spicy contrast. And honestly, you can have fun with it! This chopped salad is the perfect accompaniment for charred meats like the Yogurt-Marinated Lamb and Eggplant Kabobs (page 54) or as an additional side along with Persian Rice with Turmeric and Saffron (page 123). My advice is to eat this the same day you make it so the fruit and vegetables stay fresh and crisp. If it sits any longer, the texture changes.

2 medium Persian cucumbers, chopped into ¼-inch (6-mm) pieces, about 2 cups (210 g)

2 small-medium tomatoes, seeded and chopped into ¼-inch (6-mm) pieces, about 1 cup (180 g)

1 cup (175 g) chopped honeydew melon, cut into ¼-inch (6-mm) pieces

1 cup (150 g) chopped watermelon, cut into ¼-inch (6-mm) pieces

1 fresno pepper, chopped finely, about 2–3 tsp (15–30 g)

4 oz (113 g) feta cheese, roughly crumbled

½ cup (15 g) fresh mint leaves, chopped, plus more for garnish

⅓ cup (80 ml) olive oil

1 tbsp (15 ml) balsamic vinegar

2 tsp (10 ml) honey

Juice of ½ lemon

¼ tsp salt, or more as needed

Ground pepper

In a large bowl, add the cucumber, tomato, melons and fresno pepper and toss to combine. Top the salad with feta and mint and set aside.

In a small bowl or glass jar, whisk together the oil, vinegar, honey, lemon juice and season with salt and pepper. Taste for seasoning and pour about half of the dressing over the salad and toss everything together.

Taste for seasoning and add more dressing as needed. Garnish with mint.

 TIP: Persian cucumbers are used in this recipe because they have fewer seeds and are not as watery as traditional cucumbers. If Persian cucumbers are not available, substitute 1 long English cucumber, or if using regular cucumbers, use a spoon to scoop out the seeds.

SUMMER FRUIT AND HEIRLOOM TOMATO PANZANELLA
WITH BASIL MINT VINAIGRETTE

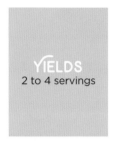

YIELDS
2 to 4 servings

I could and do eat this salad all summer long. If you know me well, you know my addiction to heirloom tomatoes. They are sweet and not nearly as acidic as their close tomato cousins, and once summer's arrival hits, I spend an obscene amount of money on heirlooms alone. My tip for the salad: ask your local bakery for some day-old bread to use. Though if the craving hits you sooner, you can toast the bread (like I've done here). Either way, the drier the bread, the better it will be able to soak up the delicious basil vinaigrette. If you'd like to make this ahead of time, arrange the tomatoes and fruit on the bottom of a large bowl and top with cubed bread, and then toss with the vinaigrette 20 minutes before serving.

CUBED BREAD

1 loaf ciabatta or French bread, cut into 1-inch (2.5-cm) pieces

2 tsp (5 g) ground sumac

2 tbsp (30 ml) olive oil

BASIL MINT VINAIGRETTE

½ cup (120 ml) olive oil

2 garlic cloves, chopped finely

1 cup (25 g) fresh mint leaves

1 cup (25 g) fresh basil leaves

1 lemon, zested and juiced

1 tsp honey

½ tsp salt

Ground pepper

SALAD

3 medium-sized heirloom tomatoes, cut into 1-inch (2.5-cm) pieces

3 stone fruit (peaches, nectarines, plums), pits removed and cut into 1-inch (2.5-cm) pieces

1 (8-oz [226-g]) ball burrata cheese

Basil and mint leaves, for garnish

Preheat the oven to 400°F (204°C) and toss the cubed bread with sumac and a good drizzle of oil on a baking sheet and bake for about 10 minutes until dried on the outside. Allow to cool to room temperature.

To make the vinaigrette, add the oil, garlic, mint, basil, lemon zest and juice, honey, salt and pepper to a food processor or blender and blend until combined. Pour vinaigrette in a small jar and set aside.

In a large bowl, toss together the tomatoes, fruit, toasted bread and enough vinaigrette so that everything is coated evenly. Arrange on a platter and gently tear the burrata cheese and place on top of the salad. Garnish with additional basil and mint leaves.

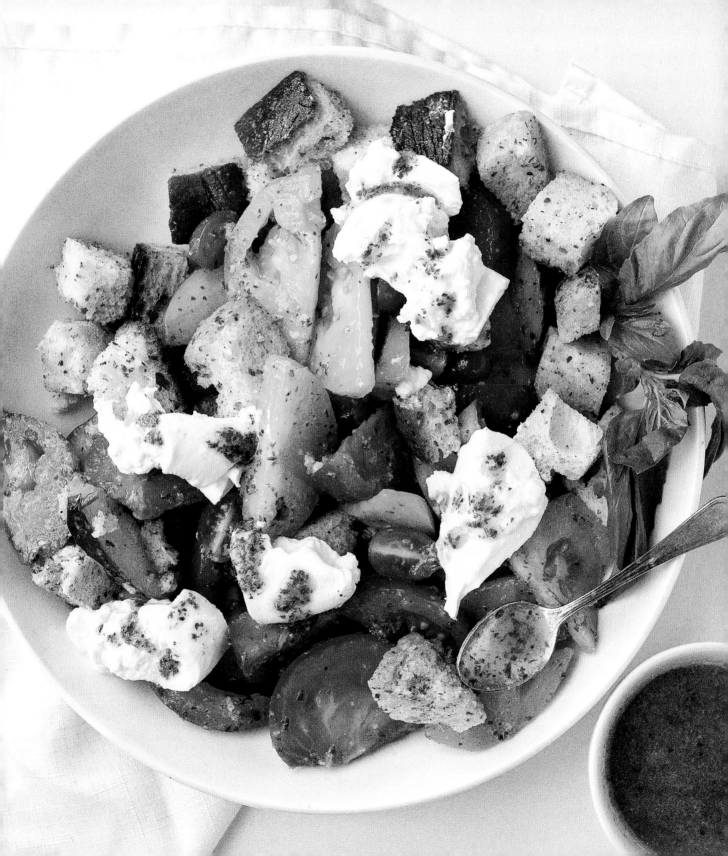

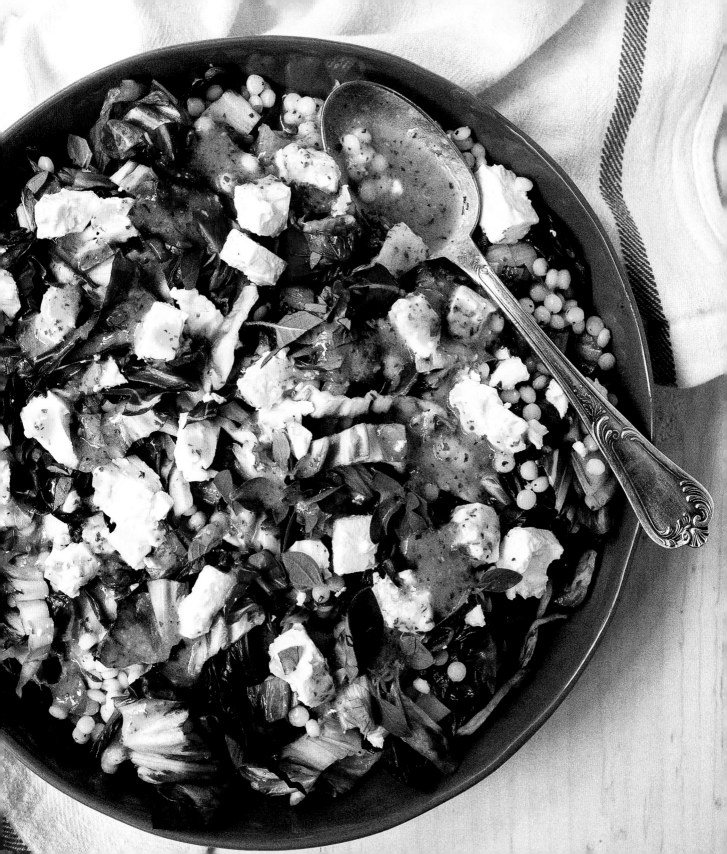

CHARRED RADICCHIO SALAD WITH ISRAELI COUSCOUS AND ANCHOVY CITRUS VINAIGRETTE

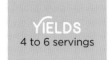

YIELDS
4 to 6 servings

Radicchio has an interesting bitter flavor that pairs wonderfully with a citrus vinaigrette. You can enjoy it raw, but when radicchio is slightly charred, the bitter taste mellows ever so gently. And don't be nervous about the anchovy vinaigrette. The small fillets break down and become a beautifully salty component that perfectly blends with the citrus flavors in the vinaigrette and smoky flavors of the charred leaves.

SALAD

8 oz (226 g) dried Israeli couscous

2 tbsp (30 ml) olive oil

2 heads radicchio, cut in quarters

1 bunch spring onions

4 oz (113 g) feta cheese, cubed

ANCHOVY CITRUS VINAIGRETTE

4 anchovy fillets

⅔ cup (160 ml) olive oil

2 garlic cloves, grated or chopped finely

4 sprigs fresh oregano, stems removed

1 lemon, zested and juiced

2 tsp (10 ml) honey

Salt and pepper, as needed

Fresh oregano leaves, for garnish

Cook the couscous according to package directions and drain. You may want to drizzle a bit of olive oil so the couscous doesn't stick together once it's cooked.

Using a grill pan on high heat, drizzle with the olive oil and char the radicchio and spring onions until the outside leaves are blistered and slightly wilted, about 2 to 3 minutes, rotating so all sides are grilled.

Remove to a cutting board and roughly chop the radicchio and spring onions. Combine with the couscous and feta.

To make the vinaigrette, add the anchovies and oil to a bowl and use a fork or whisk to break down the anchovy so it's combined well. Add the garlic, oregano, lemon zest and juice, honey and salt and pepper and whisk until combined.

Toss the salad with the vinaigrette and garnish with oregano.

CHOPPED SALAD WITH FARRO, CRISPY CHICKPEAS AND TURMERIC VINAIGRETTE

YIELDS
2 to 4 servings

I couldn't resist making another chopped salad, this one more on the savory side, full of fresh herbs, crispy baked chickpeas and chewy farro. If you're not familiar with farro, let me tell you it is a wonderful ancient grain, full of fiber and protein to keep you full and nourished.

½ cup (114 g) farro

ROASTED CHICKPEAS

1 cup (164 g) cooked chickpeas, drained and rinsed

½ tsp ground cumin

¼ tsp ground cinnamon

½ tsp ground turmeric

¼ tsp salt

2 tbsp (30 ml) olive oil

TURMERIC VINAIGRETTE

½ cup (120 ml) olive oil

2 tsp (10 ml) honey

1 tbsp (15 ml) apple cider vinegar

½ lemon, zested and juiced

1 tsp ground turmeric

¼ tsp salt, or more as needed

Ground pepper

SALAD

2 medium Persian cucumbers, chopped into ¼-inch (6-mm) pieces, about 2 cups (210 g)

4 radishes, chopped into ¼-inch (6-mm) pieces, about ½ cup (60 g)

1 medium tomato, seeded and chopped into ¼-inch (6-mm) pieces, about 1 cup (180 g)

¼ cup (45 g) pomegranate seeds

¼ cup (5 g) fresh parsley leaves, stems removed and chopped finely

¼ cup (5 g) fresh mint leaves, chopped finely

Add the farro to a small pot with 2 cups (475 ml) of water and bring to a boil. Then reduce to a constant simmer and cook for about 25 to 30 minutes. The farro should be chewy and not hard. Once done, drain and set aside.

While the farro cooks, preheat the oven to 400°F (204°C) and lay the chickpeas on a foil-lined baking sheet and dry thoroughly with a paper towel. Toss with the cumin, cinnamon, turmeric, salt and oil and bake for about 20 minutes. When done, they should be crispy with a deep brown color. Remove from the oven and set aside.

To make the vinaigrette, add the oil, honey, vinegar, lemon zest and juice, turmeric, salt and pepper to a small bowl or glass jar and whisk to combine. Taste for seasoning and adjust as needed.

In a large bowl, add the farro, cucumbers, radishes, tomatoes and pomegranate seeds and toss to combine. Add the parsley, mint and the crispy chickpeas as close to serving as possible and toss together with the vinaigrette.

 TIP: This would be great to take for weekday lunches. Layer the chopped salad in a glass jar and top with roasted chickpeas. Keep the dressing separate until you're ready to eat.

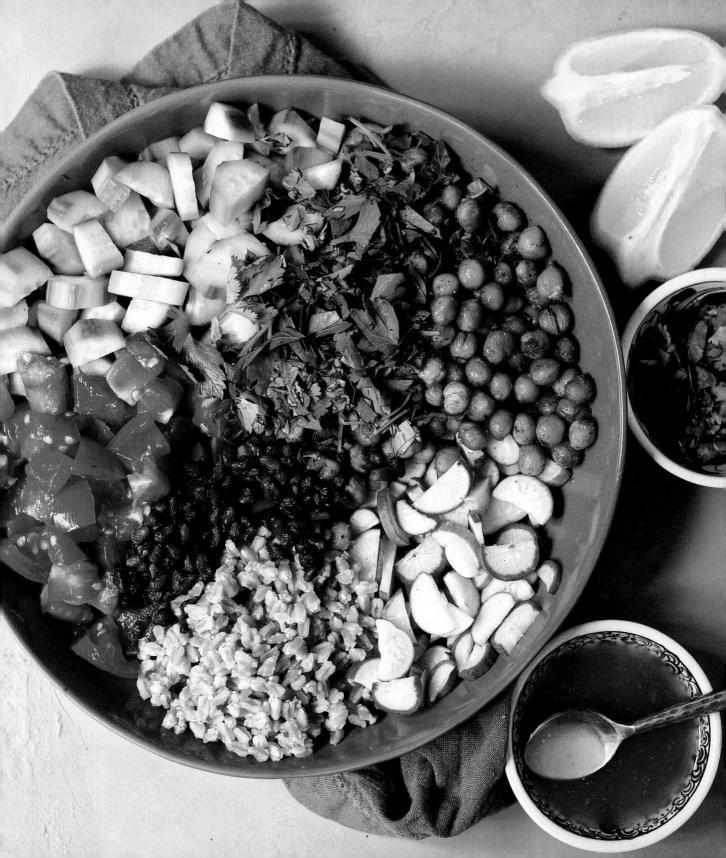

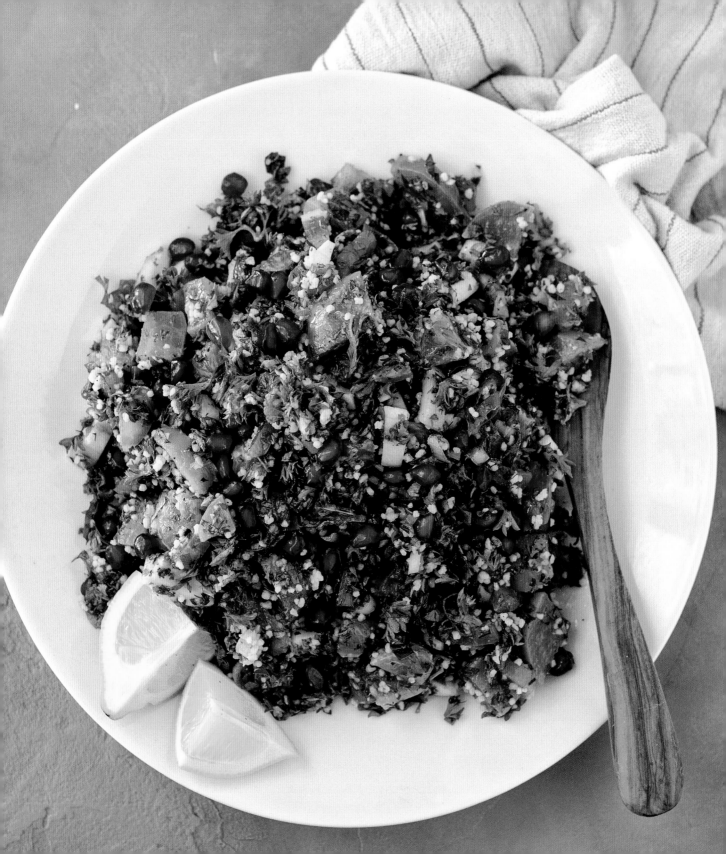

JEWELED TABBOULEH SALAD
WITH COUSCOUS

YIELDS
4 servings

This is my humble modern twist on the classic Lebanese salad. Traditionally made with bulgur, I swapped that for cooked couscous and loaded the herbaceous salad with sweet pomegranate seeds, citrus and beets. The sweetness of the fruit pairs beautifully with the tart dressing and fresh herbs.

2 medium beets

¼ cup (60 ml) olive oil

1 lemon, zested and juiced

½ tsp salt, or to taste

¼ tsp ground pepper, or to taste

½ cup (78 g) cooked couscous

1 medium-sized tomato, chopped into ¼-inch (6-mm) pieces, seeds removed

3 tangerines, peeled and cut into ¼-inch (6-mm) pieces

1 medium-sized Persian cucumber, chopped into ½-inch (1.2-cm) pieces

3 green onions, chopped

½ cup (87 g) pomegranate arils

1 cup (25 g) curly parsley, stems removed and chopped finely, about ½ bunch

¼ cup (5 g) fresh mint, stems removed and chopped

¼ cup (5 g) cilantro, stems removed and chopped

To roast the beets, preheat the oven to 400°F (204°C). Wrap the beets in foil and roast until fork tender, about 1 hour. Once done, allow them to cool enough to handle, then peel and cut into ½-inch (1.2-cm) pieces.

Make the dressing. In a bowl, whisk together the oil, lemon zest and juice, salt and pepper and set aside.

In a large bowl, add the roasted beets, couscous, tomato, tangerine, cucumber, green onions, pomegranate, parsley, mint and cilantro. Pour the dressing over the tabbouleh and gently toss everything together.

Taste for seasoning and serve immediately or place in an airtight container and chill until ready to use.

TIP: This salad holds up great for a few days and is perfect to make ahead of time. If you prefer a crispier salad, add the prepped ingredients to a large bowl and add the dressing right before serving. If you prefer a more dressed salad, toss everything together along with the dressing and cover the bowl with plastic wrap. The tabbouleh will last when dressed for up to three days.

CHOPPED RAINBOW SALAD
with CRISPY LAVASH

YIELDS
2 to 4 servings

This rainbow salad is the epitome of everything I love about big hearty salads. There's crunch, texture, freshness and a creamy yogurt dressing to round everything out. The crispy lavash holds up well, but keep it separate if you want to prolong its crunch.

2 sheets lavash bread

1 tsp garlic powder

½ tsp salt

2 tbsp (30 ml) olive oil

1 roasted beet, peeled and chopped into ½-inch (1.2-cm) pieces

2 small to medium Persian cucumbers, chopped into ½-inch (1.2-cm) pieces

1 cup (140 g) cherry tomatoes, cut in half

¾ cup (170 g) finely chopped red cabbage

1–2 radishes, sliced very thinly using a mandoline

2 green onions, chopped finely

¼ cup (5 g) fresh mint leaves, chopped

¼ cup (5 g) fresh basil leaves, chopped

YOGURT DRESSING

¼ cup (60 ml) olive oil

1 tsp mustard

2 tbsp (30 ml) full-fat Greek yogurt

5–6 scallions, chopped very finely

1 clove garlic, grated

2 tsp (10 ml) red wine vinegar

Juice of ½ lemon

Preheat the oven to 400°F (204°C) and place the lavash on a baking sheet. Sprinkle with the garlic powder, salt and olive oil and bake for about 10 minutes, until lightly golden brown and crispy. Once done, remove from the oven and break into 1-inch (2.5-cm) pieces and set aside.

In a large bowl, add together the beet, cucumber, tomatoes, cabbage, radish, green onions, mint and basil and toss to combine.

In a small bowl or glass jar, whisk together the oil, mustard, yogurt, scallions, garlic, vinegar and lemon juice. Toss about half of the dressing with the salad and crispy lavash. Add more dressing if desired and serve immediately.

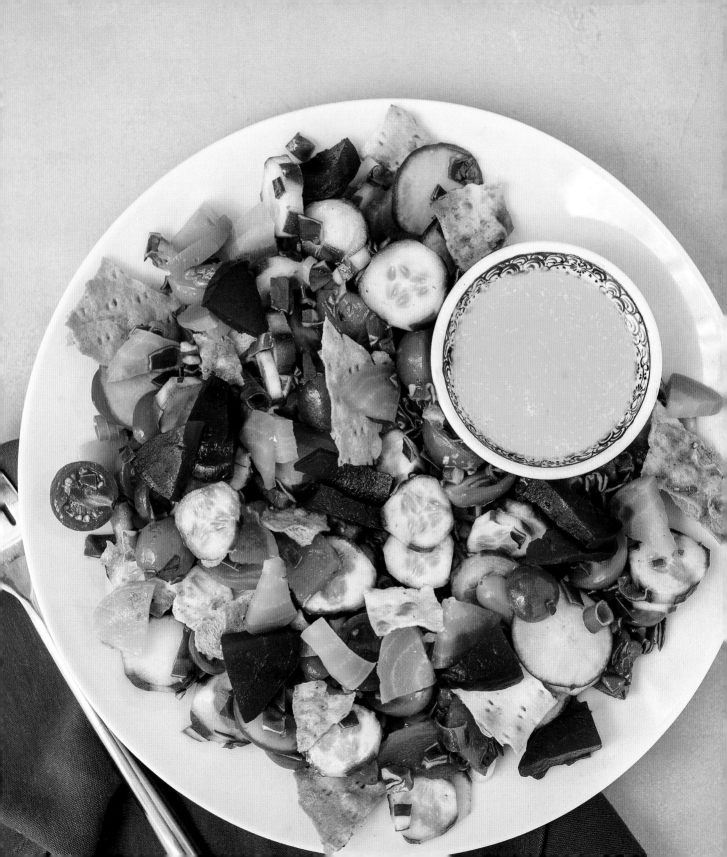

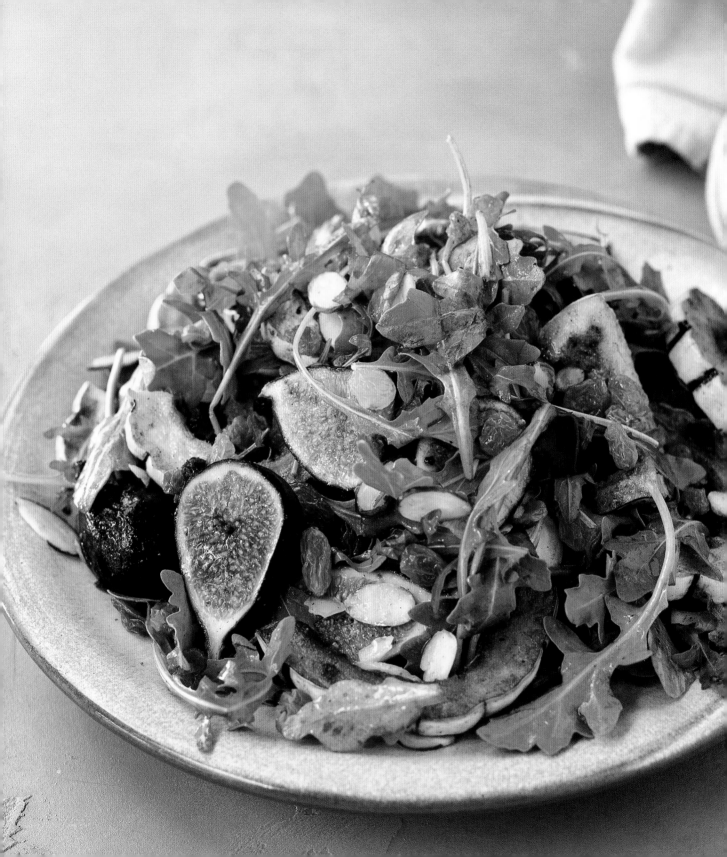

AUTUMN SQUASH SALAD
WITH FIGS AND ARUGULA

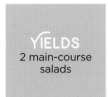

YIELDS
2 main-course salads

There is a short window of opportunity as the season slowly shifts to cooler temperatures when fresh figs are still at their peak and squash begins to ripen.

I wait impatiently every year until my favorite delicata squash is in season. The sweet nutty squash is perfect for easy weeknight meals because it needs limited prep time and roasts up beautifully. The skin is thin and sweet, so you won't need to peel anything beforehand. I promise you, this will be your new favorite squash to roast.

1 delicata squash

½ tsp ground cumin

½ tsp ground allspice

½ tsp ground cinnamon

¼ tsp salt

Ground pepper

2 tbsp (30 ml) olive oil

3 cups (75 g) baby arugula

5–6 fresh figs of any variety, cut in half

¼ cup (23 g) toasted sliced almonds

¼ cup (40 g) golden raisins

BALSAMIC VINAIGRETTE

¼ cup (60 ml) olive oil

2 tbsp (30 ml) balsamic vinegar

1 tsp Dijon mustard

1 tsp honey

¼ tsp salt

Ground pepper to taste

Preheat the oven to 400°F (204°C) and line a baking sheet with foil.

Cut the squash in half lengthwise and scoop out the seeds and discard. Slice the squash into thin half moon shapes, about ¼-inch (6-mm) thick and toss with the cumin, allspice, cinnamon, salt, pepper and olive oil. Arrange the squash in a single layer and roast for about 20 to 22 minutes or until the squash has lightly charred on the outside and softened. Once done, allow to cool for a few minutes.

In a large bowl, add together the arugula, figs, almonds, raisins and roasted squash. Make the vinaigrette by whisking together the oil, vinegar, mustard, honey, salt and pepper. Begin by dressing the salad with about half of the vinaigrette. Toss to combine and taste for seasoning; add more dressing as desired.

TIP: Anticipating the perfectly ripened fig can be nerve-racking, but it is well worth the wait. Look for figs that are soft and feel heavy for their size. The softer the fig is, the sweeter they will taste.

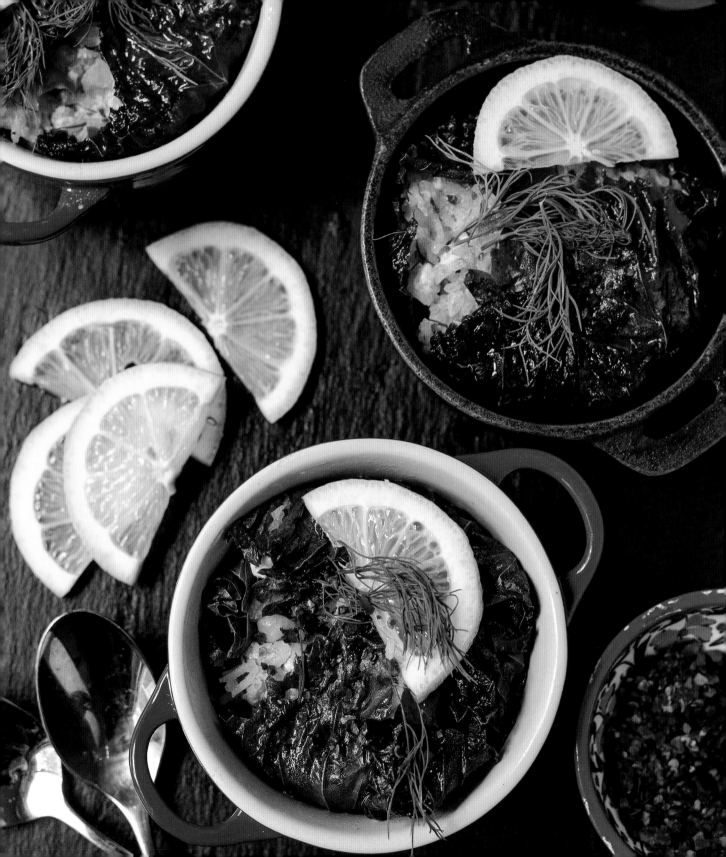

CHAPTER 4

VEGETABLES, GRAINS AND PULSES

EFFORTLESSLY HEALTHY AND WHOLESOME EATS

This is the time to raid your store's bulk bins. It's like an amusement park for me as I stand in front of all the bins, drawers and scoops. I envision so many hearty, satisfying and filling meals made with these simple and mostly ancient grains.

Rice is a necessity in Mediterranean cooking, and the cleaning and preparing of the grains is taken quite seriously. Rinse rice as much as you can to make it as airy and pillowy as possible. You can make the addictive Persian Rice with Turmeric and Saffron (page 123) that has a crispy bottom called tahdig—I'll warn you now, you'll be fighting over that crispy bottom. My other favorite grain is the hearty and satisfying farro, and personally I think it makes for an even more delicious paella in Farro Paella with Seafood and Chorizo (page 104) as it can stand up to the heat, cooks evenly and takes in all the fascinating flavors of the sauce.

Vegetables hold their own and can be the star of the show at any dinner table, and it still amazes me what mother nature can do. I have been so lucky to live in places with amazing local produce and farmers markets, so this is the time to eat seasonally to really showcase the beauty of vegetables.

Leek and Spinach Fritters with Lemon Yogurt (page 124) are near and dear to my heart as these are a play on my mom's Turkish recipe called kifticas. Roasted Cauliflower with Capers, Almonds and Pomegranate Tahini Sauce (page 120) is something made on a weekly rotation and a match made in veggie heaven. You can eat this right out of the oven, or if you manage to have any left over, it is perfect cold for a weekday lunch. But those crunchy little florets are addicting, to say the least.

Zucchini and Halloumi Rollatini (page 108) is a perfect way to use up summer's bountiful zucchini harvest. For those cooler months, sweet Harissa-Roasted Butternut Squash with Dates (page 136) is tossed with spicy harissa to make a perfect fall dish for any weeknight or even special occasion.

FARRO PAELLA WITH SEAFOOD AND CHORIZO

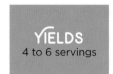

YIELDS
4 to 6 servings

Traditionally paella is made with short-grain Spanish rice, but I have found that farro creates a chewier texture and cooks more evenly. The combination of sweet tomatoes, classic saffron and spicy chorizo creates the most luxurious sauce that cooks into the farro with layers of savory flavor. Use any proteins that you have, but I love the combination of spicy smoky chorizo with fresh seafood.

2 tbsp (30 ml) olive oil

2 links Spanish chorizo, cut into ½-inch (1.2-cm) pieces

1 large shallot, diced

1 large red bell pepper, seeded and diced

3 garlic cloves, chopped finely

2 tbsp (30 ml) tomato paste

¾ tsp saffron threads

1 cup (195 g) dry farro

1 (14.5-oz [411-g]) can diced tomatoes with liquid

1½ cups (360 ml) chicken or seafood stock (or mixture of both)

½ tsp smoked paprika

¾ tsp salt, or more to taste

½ tsp ground pepper

6 medium-size whole shrimp, head-on (optional)

12–14 fresh mussels

12–14 fresh clams

¼ cup (34 g) frozen peas

¼ cup (37 g) frozen fava beans

Lemon wedges for garnish

In a 15-inch (38-cm) paella pan or large skillet, add the olive oil and place on medium-high heat. Add the chorizo and sauté until fully cooked, browning both sides, for about 3 to 4 minutes. Once done, reserve to a small plate and set aside.

Add the shallot and bell pepper and cook in the oil for 2 to 3 minutes. The shallot shouldn't brown too much, just soften. Stir in the garlic and cook for another minute.

Add the tomato paste and saffron and stir everything together, making sure the tomato paste is evenly distributed. Stir in the farro, again making sure all of the farro is coated and mixed with all the other ingredients.

Pour in the tomatoes with their juices along with the stock and season with paprika, salt and pepper. Stir everything together once more and allow the farro to settle in an even layer.

Bring to a low boil and lightly cover with a large piece of foil. This will help evenly cook everything. Depending on how large your pan and burners are, you may need to use two burners or rotate the pan every so often.

Cook until the farro is cooked through and chewy, about 25 minutes.

Once the farro is cooked, nestle in the shrimp, mussels and clams and add back in the chorizo. Cover again with foil and cook until the shrimp is opaque and the mussels and clams have opened, about 10 to 12 minutes.

Turn off the heat and scatter in the peas and fava beans. Cover with foil again and allow the steam to warm up the peas and fava beans for another 2 to 3 minutes. Serve with lemon wedges.

 TIP: This is one of those versatile meals where you can play around with flavors and ingredients. If you can't find fava beans, use all peas. If clams aren't in season, use mussels or all shrimp. Either way, it will all be delicious.

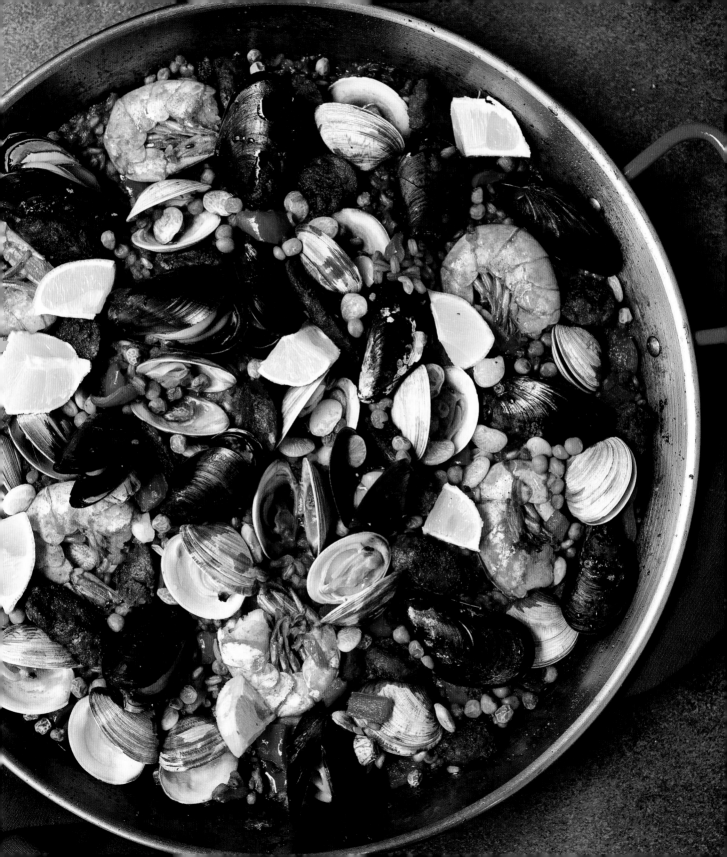

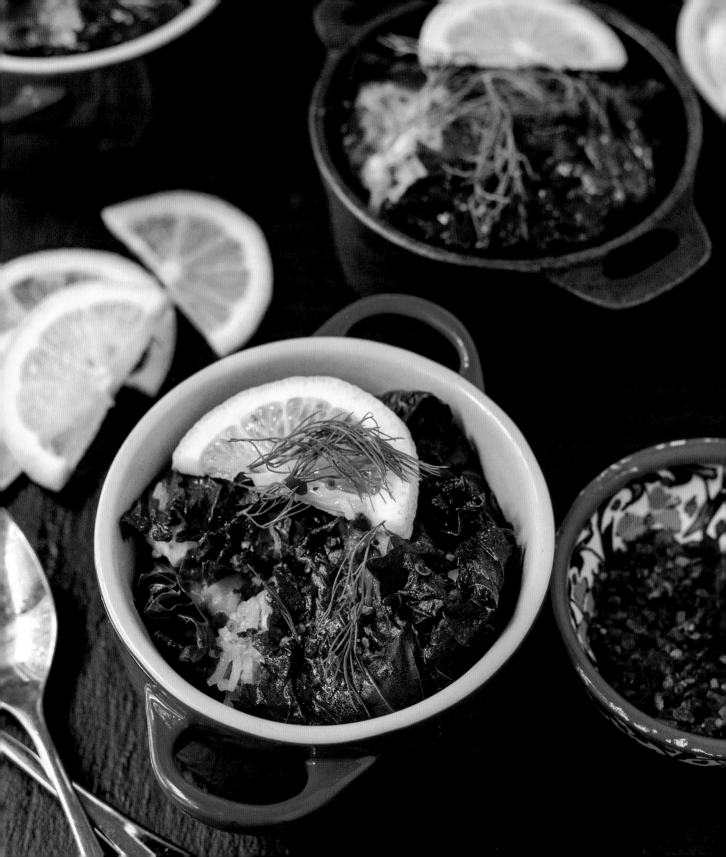

UNSTUFFED GRAPE LEAVES

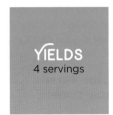

YIELDS
4 servings

One of my first cooking memories is rolling grape leaves. It's a rewarding process but does take a long, long time. Here I created a much easier way to enjoy all the same flavors. Instead of rolling each individual grape leaf, lay them in a small casserole dish and fill. This can also be done with any size casserole dish, but I think the smaller ones are just so cute!

These would be great with a dollop of Magical Herb Tahini Sauce (page 147) or Cucumber, Yogurt and Mint Dip (page 160).

12–16 medium-large jarred grape leaves

3 tbsp (45 ml) olive oil, divided

½ cup (80 g) finely chopped red onion

1 red bell pepper, seeded and chopped into ¼-inch (6-mm) pieces

2 garlic cloves, chopped finely

1 medium tomato, chopped into ½-inch (1.2-cm) pieces

4 fresh oregano sprigs, stems removed and leaves chopped

4 fresh dill sprigs, stems removed and leaves chopped

½ tsp Aleppo pepper flakes

Salt, to taste

½ tsp dried mint

Zest of 1 lemon

1 cup (200 g) cooked basmati rice

1 cup (210 g) canned chickpeas

6 oz (170 g) cubed feta cheese

Preheat the oven to 350°F (176°C).

Remove the grape leaves from the jar and rinse under cool water, separating each leaf. Pat them dry and set aside.

In a small pot over medium heat, add 1 tablespoon (15 ml) of oil, the onion and bell pepper and sauté for 3 to 4 minutes until just softened.

Add the garlic and cook for another minute, and then add the tomatoes, oregano, dill, Aleppo pepper, salt, mint and lemon zest and cook for another 2 minutes so the tomatoes can release their juices. Taste for seasoning and set aside.

In a large bowl combine the cooked rice, chickpeas and feta cheese and pour in the tomato mixture, mixing everything together.

Brush a generous layer of oil all over the inside of four 8-ounce (240-ml) casserole dishes or one 8-inch by 8-inch (20 × 20-cm) casserole dish. Lay 3 to 4 leaves inside each dish, overlapping so there are no gaps and leaving a 1-inch (2.5-cm) overhang.

Fill each dish with stuffing and fold over the edges of grape leaves. Brush 1 tablespoon (15 ml) of olive oil on top of the grape leaves and bake for 15 to 18 minutes until the tops of the leaves are darkened in color and slightly crispy.

Remove from the oven and allow to cool for 5 minutes before serving.

ZUCCHINI AND HALLOUMI ROLLATINI

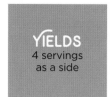

YIELDS
4 servings
as a side

This is for when summer's zucchini is at its peak, and you're scrambling to find new recipe ideas to use up the garden's bounty. You'll be able to find halloumi cheese (feta's not-as-salty and firmer cousin) in many specialty and international stores, however if you can't, substitute a good-quality feta cheese.

Serve on the side with Basmati Rice with Pistachios, Lima Beans and Dill (page 119) and Yogurt-Marinated Lamb and Eggplant Kabobs (page 54) for a fully delectable dinner.

2 lbs (907 g) zucchini, sliced thin using a mandoline

Salt, as needed

Olive oil, as needed

2 garlic cloves, chopped finely

1 tsp dried mint

2 medium tomatoes, seeded and chopped

1 lemon, juiced and zested

Pepper, to taste

8 oz (226 g) halloumi cheese, cut into ½-inch (1.2-cm) cubes

Fresh mint and chives, roughly chopped for garnish

Preheat the oven to 400°F (260°C).

Lay the zucchini slices on a parchment-lined baking sheet. Sprinkle with a pinch of salt and place them in the oven for 10 minutes. This will help soften the slices so they are easier to roll.

While the zucchini is baking, make the tomato sauce. In a small pot on medium heat, drizzle olive oil and add garlic and sauté until lightly golden, about 2 to 3 minutes. Add the dried mint and stir thoroughly.

Add the tomatoes with juices and the lemon juice and zest. Season with salt and pepper and adjust as necessary. Cook for another 3 minutes so the tomatoes break down a bit and the flavors blend. Once done, pour the sauce into a medium-sized 9-inch x 6-inch (22.8-cm x 15.2-cm) baking dish and set aside.

Remove the zucchini from the oven and allow to cool enough to handle. Place a cube of halloumi cheese at the end of a zucchini slice and roll it up. Arrange the zucchini rollups in the baking dish on top of the sauce, drizzle the rollups with oil and place back in the oven for another 10 minutes.

Remove from the oven and garnish with mint and chives. The zucchini should be tender but not overcooked and the cheese slightly melted and softened.

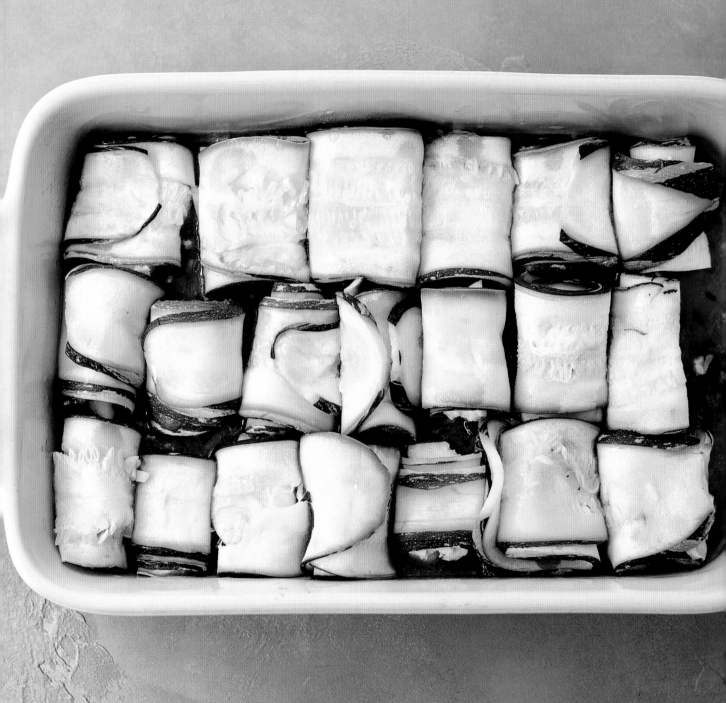

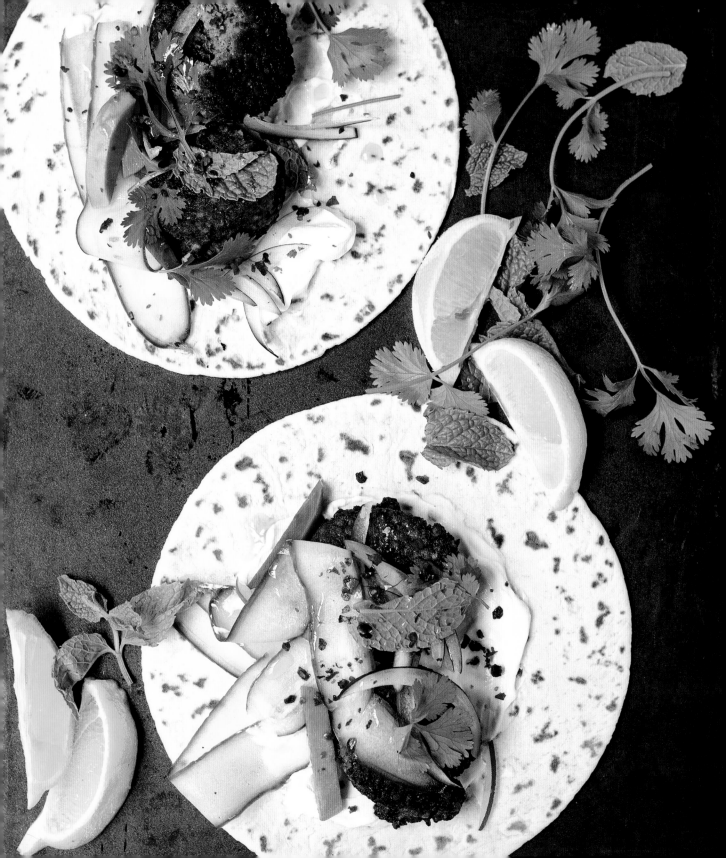

RED LENTIL FALAFEL

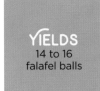

YIELDS
14 to 16
falafel balls

I don't fry often, but when I do, it's always for falafel. You need to plan well to make the traditional dried bean falafel, which requires soaking the beans overnight. Instead, this lentil falafel is a spin-off from the traditional with all the same flavors and a fraction of the soaking time. Falafel is fabulous to add to a multitude of dishes. Use falafel to top your favorite salad, stuff inside a pita pocket or wrap with tender butter lettuce. Serve falafel with Cucumber, Yogurt and Mint Dip (page 160) or Magical Herb Tahini Sauce (page 147) either drizzled over or on the side to dip.

1 cup (200 g) dried red lentils

½ cup (12 g) fresh parsley, hard stems removed

½ cup (12 g) fresh cilantro, stems removed

1 shallot, roughly chopped

2 garlic cloves, roughly chopped

1 tsp ground turmeric

1 tsp ground cumin

½ tsp cayenne

Zest of 1 lemon

1 tbsp (15 ml) lemon juice

½ tsp baking soda

1 tsp baking powder

2 tbsp (15 g) flour (all-purpose or chickpea will work)

Canola or vegetable oil for frying

¼ tsp salt, plus more for garnish, if needed

Cucumber, Yogurt and Mint Dip (page 160) or Magical Herb Tahini Sauce (page 147), for serving

Add the lentils to a large bowl and quickly sort through them, picking out any stones or discolored lentils. Pour in enough room temperature water to completely cover the lentils and soak for about 1 hour. The lentils will expand to about 3 times their original size.

Drain the lentils and add to a food processor. Blend to a coarse crumble that is not mushy or soft and transfer to a large bowl.

In the same food processor add the parsley, cilantro, shallot, garlic, turmeric, cumin, cayenne, lemon zest and juice. Blend together to a coarse consistency. Use a small spatula to scrape down the sides if needed, as you don't want any large pieces left over. Once done, add to the lentils along with the baking soda, baking powder and flour and mix everything together until well combined.

Heat a large skillet with ½ inch (1.2 cm) of oil until it reaches about 360°F (182°C). Using wet hands, if needed, scoop out a heaping tablespoon (15 ml) of mixture, rounding it into a flat ball and gently placing it in the hot oil. Fry the first side for about 3 to 4 minutes until you can see it begin to brown up the sides, and then flip over and cook the other side for another 2 minutes.

Continue with the rest of the batter, frying no more than 4 to 5 falafel at a time. As they are done, transfer the hot falafel to a paper towel–lined baking sheet and sprinkle with a pinch of salt while they are hot.

Serve immediately alongside yogurt or tahini sauce.

 TIP: If you don't have a thermometer to test the oil temperature, place a small piece of batter into the oil and if it sizzles right away, it's ready.

TURMERIC LEMON COUSCOUS
WITH CURRANTS

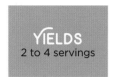

YIELDS
2 to 4 servings

A staple in the pantry, couscous is inexpensive and easy to cook. This is where you can really get creative, using different spices and dried fruit. The simple yet vivid colors of turmeric and pomegranate seeds really make this humble pasta pop! Serve alongside Pomegranate-Glazed Lamb Chops (page 61) or Olive Oil-Braised Chicken with Fennel and Citrus (page 57).

3 tbsp (45 ml) olive oil

1 small shallot, chopped finely

1 garlic clove, chopped finely

1 tsp ground turmeric

1 cup (240 ml) vegetable or chicken stock

⅔ cup (115 g) dried couscous

1 lemon, zested and juiced

½ cup (72 g) currants

Pomegranate seeds, for garnish

Finely chopped cilantro leaves, for garnish

Place a pot on medium heat and drizzle with olive oil. Add the shallot and cook until it begins to caramelize, about 2 to 3 minutes.

Add the garlic and turmeric and continue sautéing until it is lightly golden, about another minute.

Pour in the stock and bring to a boil. Once boiling, remove the pot from the heat and add the couscous, lemon zest and juice and stir once with a spoon. Add the currants on top, cover with a lid and allow to sit for 10 minutes. Once done, fluff the couscous with a fork and garnish with pomegranate seeds and cilantro.

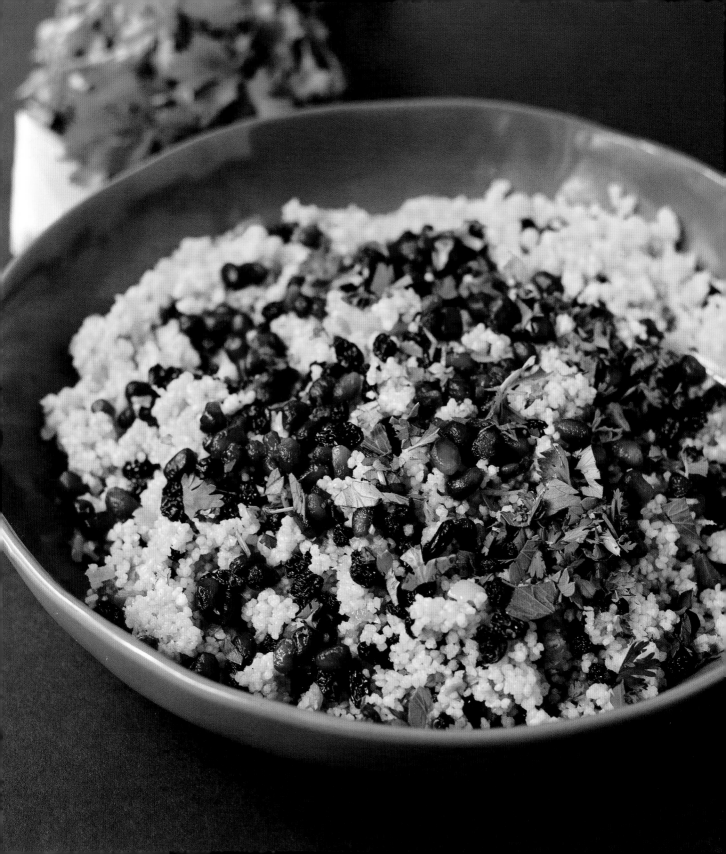

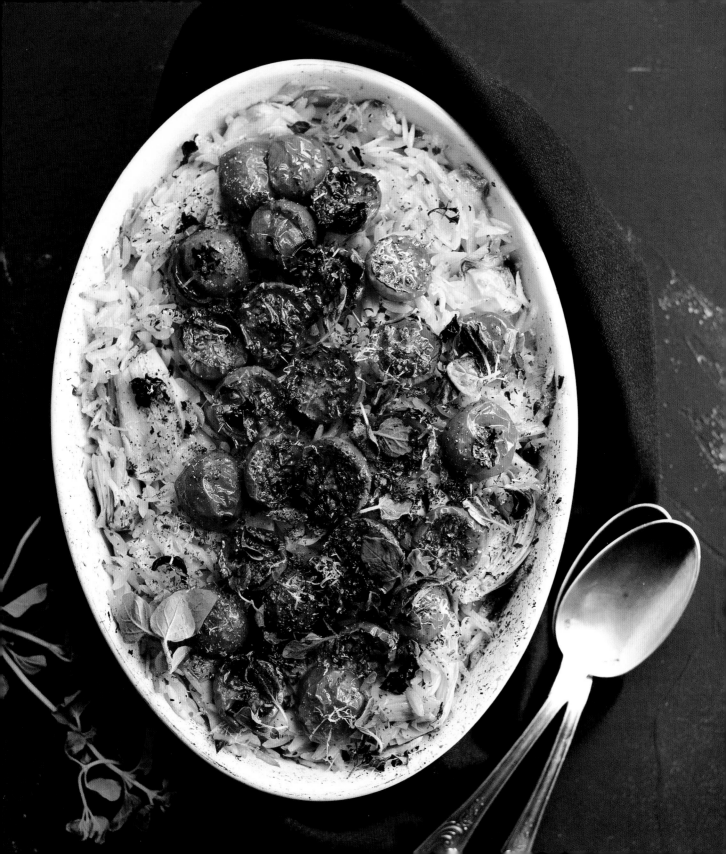

BAKED ORZO WITH ARTICHOKES, TOMATOES AND HALLOUMI

YIELDS
4 servings

This is one of those dishes where pantry staples become lifesavers. Throw it all together, bake and dinner is served. This baked orzo lasts for a few days and tastes great right out of the oven, or cold for a quick lunch. If you can't find halloumi, feta is a nice substitute.

8 oz (226 g) dried orzo

2 tbsp (30 ml) olive oil, plus 1 tsp, divided

3 garlic cloves, chopped finely

1 tsp Aleppo pepper flakes

Zest of 1 lemon

15 oz (425 g) canned or frozen and thawed artichoke hearts, cut in half

8 oz (226 g) halloumi cheese, cut in small cubes

4 oz (113 g) grated Parmesan cheese, divided

4 oz (113 g) cherry or grape tomatoes, cut in half

1 tsp dried oregano

Salt, as needed

Preheat the oven to 400°F (204°C) and bring a pot of water to a boil. Add in the orzo and cook until just about done, about 7 to 8 minutes. Once done, drain the orzo and set aside.

In a small pan, heat 2 tablespoons (30 ml) of oil and add the garlic, Aleppo pepper, lemon zest and artichoke hearts and sauté until the garlic is lightly caramelized, about 2 minutes. Add the artichoke mixture to the cooked orzo, along with the halloumi and Parmesan, and toss everything together. Add salt and taste for seasoning.

Transfer the mixture to an oiled 12-inch by 8½-inch (30 × 21-cm) casserole dish (or one of similar size) and top with cherry tomatoes, dried oregano and an extra grating of Parmesan cheese. Drizzle the remaining olive oil on top and bake for 20 minutes until the tomatoes begin to lightly char and get soft.

Allow to cool for 5 minutes before serving.

BEET-INFUSED ISRAELI COUSCOUS WITH BEET VINAIGRETTE

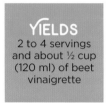
YIELDS
2 to 4 servings and about ½ cup (120 ml) of beet vinaigrette

You may want to slather this beet vinaigrette onto everything you eat, and especially toss it with Israeli couscous. The couscous soaks up the gorgeous beet flavors and turns the dish the most beautiful eye-catching shade of rose. To make prepping even quicker, roast the two beets ahead of time! Wash the beets well and cut the larger ones in half, and then wrap in foil and roast at 400°F (204°C) for about 45 minutes or until tender (the time may vary based on size). Once cool, peel and keep in an airtight container in the fridge until ready to use.

BEET VINAIGRETTE

1 small roasted beet, chopped

¼ cup (60 ml) olive oil

1 lemon, zested and juiced

1 tbsp (15 ml) balsamic vinegar

1 tbsp (7 g) za'atar

¼ tsp salt

Ground pepper

BEET-INFUSED COUSCOUS

2 tbsp (30 ml) olive oil

1 garlic clove, chopped finely

1 bunch beet greens, stems removed and chopped

¼ cup (5 g) loosely packed mint leaves, chopped

¼ tsp salt

2 tbsp (18 g) currants or raisins

1 cup dried Israeli couscous

1 roasted beet, chopped

¼ cup (34 g) toasted pine nuts

¼ cup (38 g) crumbled feta cheese

Make the beet vinaigrette. In a food processor or blender. Add the roasted beet, oil, lemon zest and juice, vinegar, za'atar, salt and pepper and blend until smooth.

In a skillet over medium heat, drizzle in the oil and add the garlic. Sauté the garlic until it is lightly caramelized, about 1 to 2 minutes. Add in the beet greens, mint and salt and continue cooking until the beet greens have wilted. Stir in the currants and set aside.

Boil the couscous in a pot filled with water until fully cooked through, about 8 to 10 minutes. Once done, drain and toss with the vinaigrette. Top the couscous with sautéed beet greens, roasted beets, pine nuts and feta.

TIP: Both the beet and beet greens are used in this recipe, so the next time you buy a bunch of beets, save those greens and use them as you would spinach or any other leafy green. If you don't have beet greens, feel free to substitute baby spinach or lacinato kale.

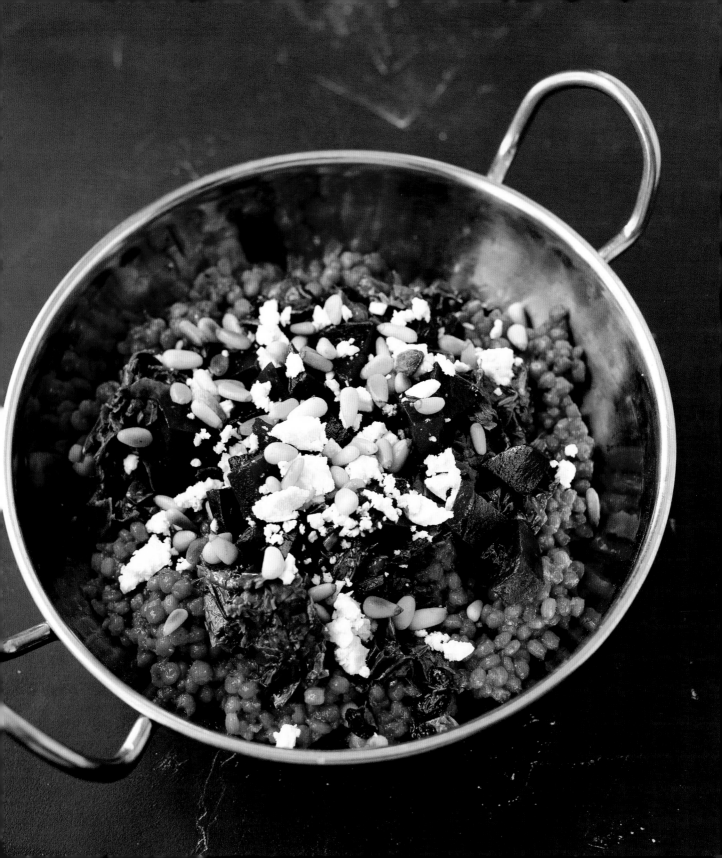

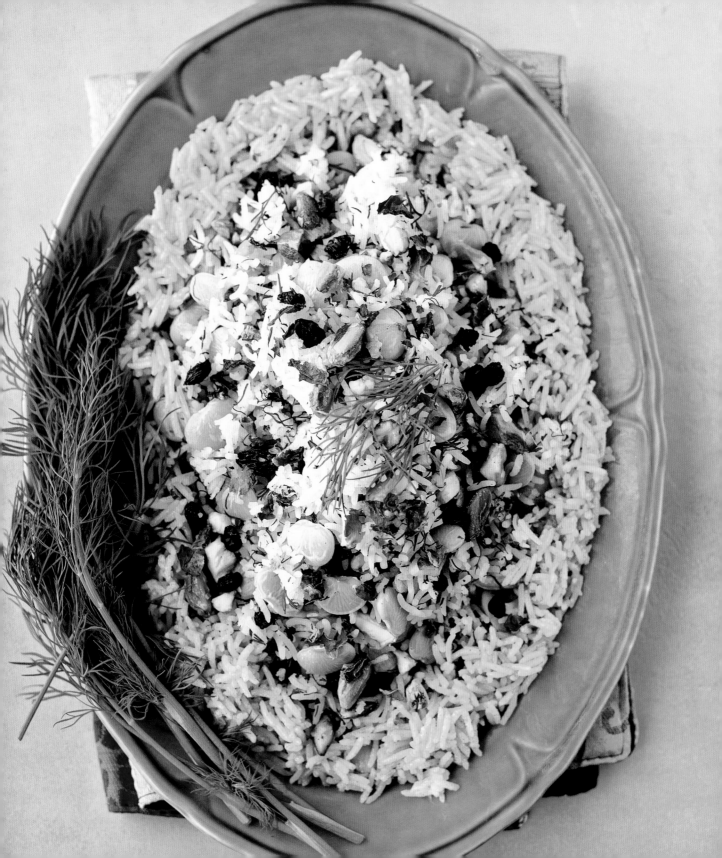

BASMATI RICE WITH PISTACHIOS, LIMA BEANS AND DILL

YIELDS
2 servings

Pistachios and dill make for such fragrant rice, and lima beans add a wonderful texture. Stir a portion of the rice with some saffron to create a beautiful plate with an added aromatic layer of flavor. Feel free to substitute fava beans or chickpeas for the lima beans for added textural contrast.

1 cup (185 g) basmati rice

½ tsp salt

2 tbsp (30 ml) olive oil

1 cup (178 g) frozen or cooked lima beans

¼ tsp saffron, finely ground

1 tbsp (15 ml) water

1 tbsp (14 g) softened butter

½ cup (62 g) pistachios, roughly chopped

¼ cup (36 g) currants or raisins

¼ cup (5 g) fresh dill, roughly chopped, plus more for garnish

2 tbsp (3 g) rose petals, for garnish (optional)

Rinse the rice under water several times until the water runs clear. Add it to a water-filled pot along with the salt and bring to a gentle boil.

Cook the rice until it's half-cooked, about 6 to 8 minutes. The outside should be tender but the middle still hard. Drain the rice and set aside.

In the same pot, add the olive oil and place the rice back into the pot along with the lima beans. Use chopsticks or a spoon handle and make several holes in the rice. Tightly tie a clean kitchen towel around the lid and cover the pot. Cook the rice for another 10 minutes until it is cooked through.

In a small bowl, stir together the saffron and water and steep for a few minutes and set aside.

Once the rice is done, transfer ¼ cup (40 g) of the cooked rice into a small bowl and stir together with the saffron water and butter. This will color the rice and give it an extra layer of flavor.

Add the pistachios, currants and dill to the rest of the rice and transfer to a platter. Garnish with the saffron-colored rice around the perimeter and scatter rose petals and fresh dill over the top.

 TIP: In this recipe I use an interesting technique of covering the lid with a clean kitchen towel. This is to prevent excess condensation from dripping onto the cooked rice and making it sticky. The towel absorbs the moisture, creating airy and separated rice.

ROASTED CAULIFLOWER WITH CAPERS, ALMONDS AND POMEGRANATE TAHINI SAUCE

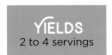
YIELDS
2 to 4 servings

Not just a vegetable side, spiced, roasted cauliflower can play along with any mezze platter and be the star of the show. Unlike its close fried Lebanese cousin, these florets are roasted on high heat to get that crispy crunch. Dip into creamy tahini sauce with a good drizzle of pomegranate molasses and end it all with a fresh squeeze of lemon juice.

1 large cauliflower, about 2 lb (907 g), cut into small florets

1 tsp ground cumin

2 tsp (5 g) ground turmeric

¾ tsp salt, divided

2 tbsp (30 ml) olive oil

2 tbsp (17 g) capers

¼ cup (23 g) sliced almonds

½ cup (120 ml) tahini

¼ cup (60 ml) water, as needed to thin out consistency

Juice of ½ lemon

1 tbsp (15 ml) pomegranate molasses

¼ cup (5 g) chopped parsley or cilantro

Lemon wedges, for serving

Preheat the oven to 425°F (218°C) and line a baking sheet with foil.

Toss the cauliflower florets with the cumin, turmeric, ½ teaspoon of salt and olive oil and roast for about 10 to 15 minutes.

Remove the pan from the oven and scatter the capers and sliced almonds onto the cauliflower and continue roasting everything for another 8 to 10 minutes.

The cauliflower should be a light golden brown with crispy edges and the almonds should be toasted.

In a small bowl, whisk together the tahini, water, lemon juice and ¼ teaspoon salt. Continue whisking until you achieve a smooth consistency. Transfer this mixture to a bowl and top with a drizzle of pomegranate molasses.

Garnish the cauliflower with parsley and serve alongside the tahini sauce and lemon wedges.

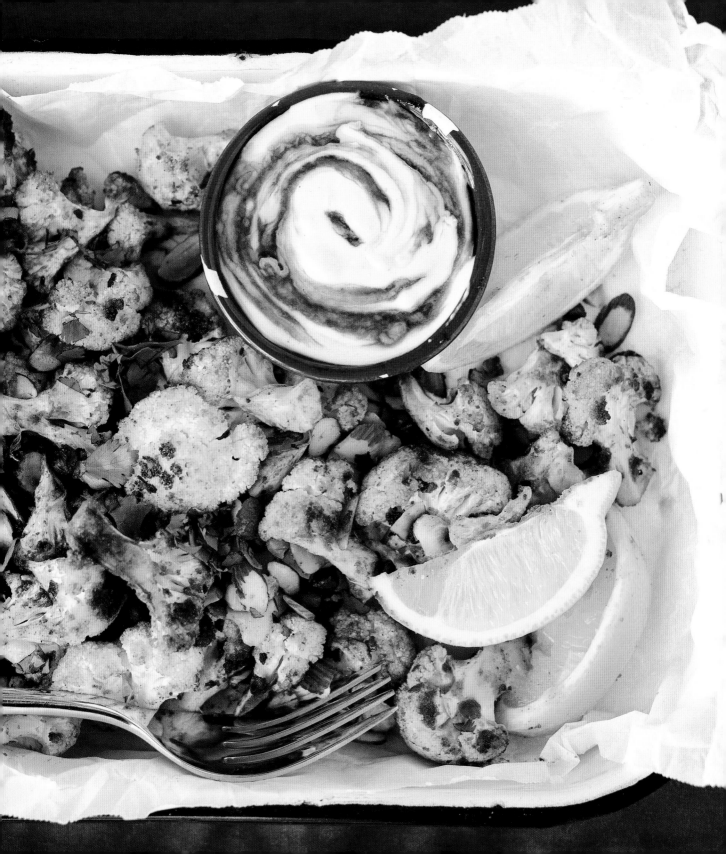

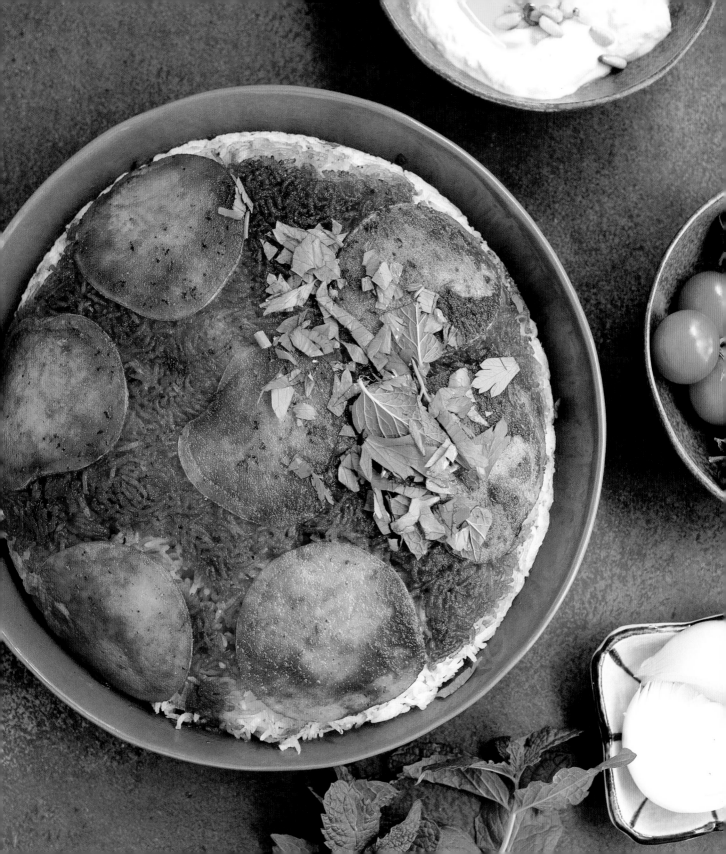

PERSIAN RICE WITH TURMERIC AND SAFFRON

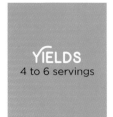

YIELDS
4 to 6 servings

Learning to make Persian tahdig is one of my most prized memories. Tahdig is the Persian word for bottom of the pot, or "tah" meaning bottom and "dig" meaning pot. It is the addictive crispy-rice bottom that many literally fight over.

My best friend's Persian boyfriend taught me to soak the rice at least overnight, but on a weeknight, the craving for Persian rice is a strong one. The flavors are simple but pronounced and both the turmeric and saffron create the most alluring golden hue against the crispy potato bottom. Serve alongside Pomegranate-Glazed Lamb Chops (page 61) or Everyday Chicken Shawarma (page 62).

2 cups (370 g) basmati rice

½ tsp salt

¼ tsp saffron, crushed

1 tbsp (15 ml) warm water

3 tbsp (45 ml) olive oil

1 tsp ground turmeric

1 Yukon gold potato, sliced very thin using a mandoline

Rinse the rice several times until the water runs clear. This will help the rice become light and aerated and not as starchy as traditional rice. Fill a large pot with water and add the salt and the rice. Bring to a gentle boil and cook the rice for about half the time as the package says, about 6 to 8 minutes.

Check the rice for doneness by squeezing one between your fingers. If it's soft on the outside and still hard on the inside, it's ready. Drain the rice in a colander, but do not rinse. Set aside.

In a small bowl, stir together the saffron and water and steep for a few minutes.

Place a 13- to 15-inch (33- to 38-cm) non-stick skillet over medium-high heat and add the olive oil, turmeric and saffron water. Add the sliced potatoes and toss everything to coat evenly and cook the potatoes for 2 to 3 minutes to give them a head start. Arrange the potato slices in a single even layer on the bottom of the pan.

Carefully add the rice to the pan, making sure the entire bottom is covered with rice. Use a toothpick or spoon handle and make 3 to 4 small holes in the rice.

Tightly tie a clean kitchen towel around the lid and cover the pan. The towel will help absorb excess moisture so the rice stays light and separated.

Continue cooking the rice for about 25 to 30 minutes until you can hear crackling sounds.

Once done, turn off the heat and either invert the rice onto a platter as whole or scoop the rice onto a platter and then use a flat spatula to remove the crispy potato tandig from the pot and serve the crispy parts on the side.

TIPS: Soaked rice is preferred for this recipe. However, rinsing the rice several times until clear water is visible is just as good. But if you do have the time and remember to soak it before you go to sleep, by all means, do so.

Use a non-stick skillet as it will help the crispy bottom not stick too much to the pan.

LEEK AND SPINACH FRITTERS WITH LEMON YOGURT

YIELDS
9 to 10 fritters

Also called kifticas or keftes, these are Sephardic leek patties. My mom always made hers thick like a hamburger patty, however I prefer the kifticas simply thin, lightly fried and full of leeks. A sprinkle of warm spices is added to the batter as my personal modern take and blends beautifully with the oniony flavors.

The batter is wet, but don't let that alarm you; as they fry they become golden, crispy and deliciously savory.

2–3 tbsp (30–45 ml) grape-seed oil

2 cups (320 g) chopped leeks, white and light green parts only, cleaned well

1 cup (150 g) frozen chopped spinach, defrosted or cooked and cooled fresh spinach

3 whole eggs

1 tbsp (15 g) breadcrumbs

1 tsp ground cumin

½ tsp ground turmeric

Pinch of cayenne

¼ tsp kosher salt

1 lemon, zested and juiced

½ cup (120 ml) full-fat Greek yogurt

Freshly chopped cilantro, for garnish

In a frying pan, add enough grape-seed oil to lightly coat the bottom. Add the leeks and cook on medium heat until just wilted, about 5 minutes, stirring continually so they don't burn. Once done, turn off the heat and set aside.

Squeeze out any excess moisture from the defrosted spinach, which will ensure a good crisp fry. In a large bowl, add the spinach, leeks, eggs, breadcrumbs, cumin, turmeric, cayenne and salt and whisk everything together until well combined.

Add a bit more oil into the same frying pan if needed and pour a heaping tablespoon (15 ml) of batter into the oil. Cook for about 1 to 2 minutes until golden brown and use a thin spatula to carefully flip the fritter over and cook for an additional minute until golden brown.

Depending how large your skillet is, you can fit 3 to 4 fritters at once. Once done, remove to a paper towel–lined plate.

To make the yogurt sauce, simply whisk together the lemon zest and juice with the yogurt.

Garnish the fritters with fresh cilantro and serve with lemon yogurt.

 TIP: These are just as delicious at room temperature and will keep in the fridge for up to 2 days.

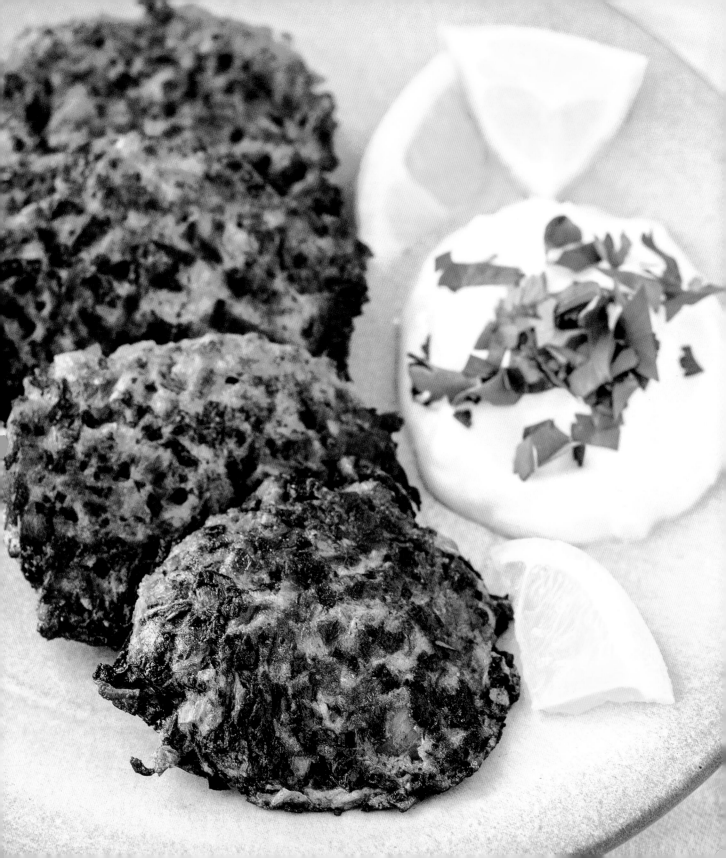

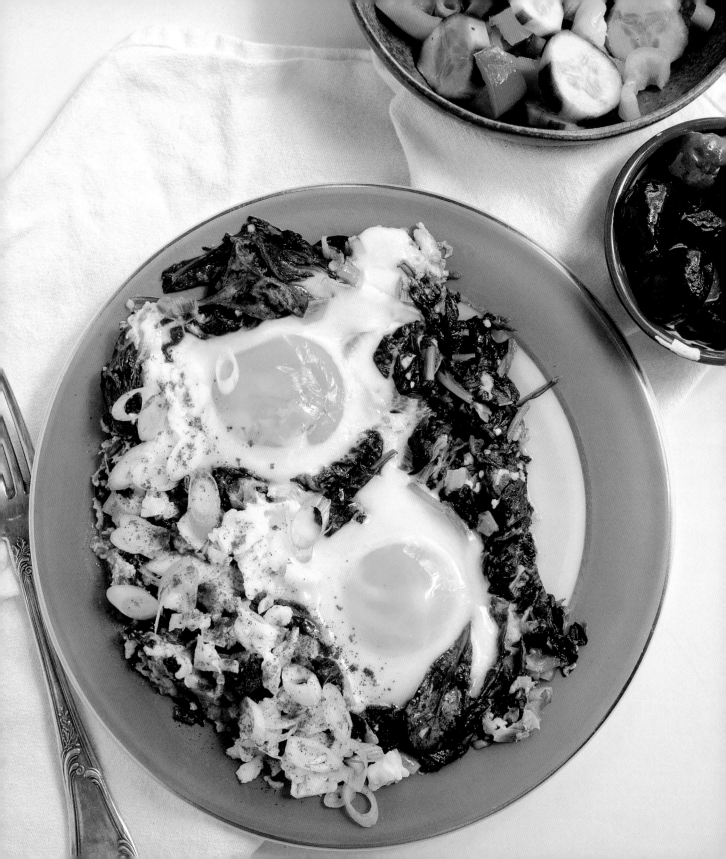

TURKISH EGGS WITH SPINACH AND YOGURT

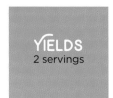

YIELDS
2 servings

This is my rustic take on Turkish eggs with yogurt. The poached version is called cilbir in Turkish and is a wonderful savory breakfast. Leeks and spinach are quickly sautéed and mixed together with creamy Greek yogurt. The eggs are poached ever-so-gently in a little nest.

Serve with toasted bread because you'll want to sop up the runny yolk and creamy spinach. For a truly delicious Turkish breakfast, serve with olives and tomatoes on the side.

2 tbsp (30 ml) olive oil

1 large leek, white and light green parts thinly sliced and cleaned well

4 cups (100 g) fresh baby spinach

2 tbsp (30 ml) 2% or full-fat Greek yogurt

4 eggs

1 green onion, chopped finely

½ tsp ground sumac

½ tsp Aleppo pepper flakes

¼ tsp salt

Heat a 10-inch (25-cm) non-stick skillet over medium heat and add the oil and leek. Sauté the leek until wilted, about 3 to 5 minutes.

Add in the spinach and cook until the spinach cooks down for another 1 to 2 minutes.

Reduce the heat to low and stir in the yogurt, so it coats the vegetables.

Use the back of a spoon or spatula to make 4 wells. Carefully crack one egg into each indented well.

Continue cooking until the egg whites are set, about 5 to 6 minutes. Cover with a lid to help cook the tops of the eggs if needed.

Once done, turn off the heat and garnish with green onions, sumac, Aleppo pepper and salt.

 TIP: This is another perfect recipe for frozen spinach; just make sure to squeeze out any excess moisture.

MEDITERRANEAN RATATOUILLE
WITH PISTACHIO PESTO

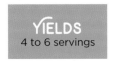

YIELDS
4 to 6 servings

This is a very modern and simple play on the classic French version with the addition of my favorite vegetable—roasted fennel. Unlike in its raw state, roasted fennel becomes caramelized and takes on a totally different mild and sweet flavor profile. Serve with crusty bread and a bright pistachio pesto.

RATATOUILLE

2 lbs (907 g) green zucchini, sliced in ½-inch (1.2-cm) rounds

1 sweet onion, sliced thin

1 small eggplant, cut into ½-inch (1.2-cm) cubes

2 bell peppers, cut into ½-inch (1.2-cm) strips

1 fennel bulb, core removed and sliced into ½-inch (1.2-cm) strips

8 oz (226 g) cherry tomatoes

1 whole garlic head, cut in half

2 tsp (4 g) dried mint

1½ tsp (5 g) za'atar

1 tsp Aleppo pepper flakes

½ tsp garlic powder

Salt, as needed

Olive oil, as needed

Chopped pistachios, for garnish

PISTACHIO PESTO

6 oz (170 g) shelled pistachios

2 oz (56 g) grated Parmesan

½ cup (120 ml) olive oil

1 lemon, zest and juice

Small bunch fresh mint, stems removed

Small bunch fresh basil, stems removed

Preheat the oven to 400°F (204°C).

Toss the zucchini, onion, eggplant, peppers, fennel, tomatoes and garlic on a foil-lined baking sheet with the mint, za'atar, Aleppo pepper, garlic powder, salt and a drizzle of olive oil. Arrange the vegetables in an even single layer and bake for 35 to 40 minutes until the vegetables are tender.

To make the pesto, add the pistachios, Parmesan, oil, lemon zest and juice, mint and basil to a food processor and blend until the desired consistency.

Remove the vegetables from the oven and garnish with pistachios and pistachio pesto.

The pistachio pesto will keep in an airtight container in the fridge for up to 5 days.

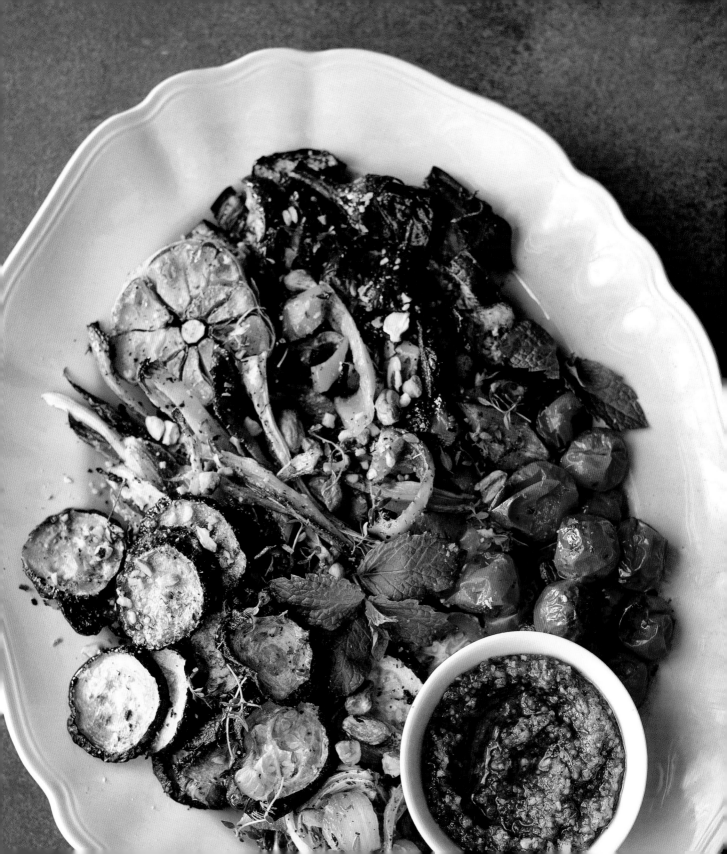

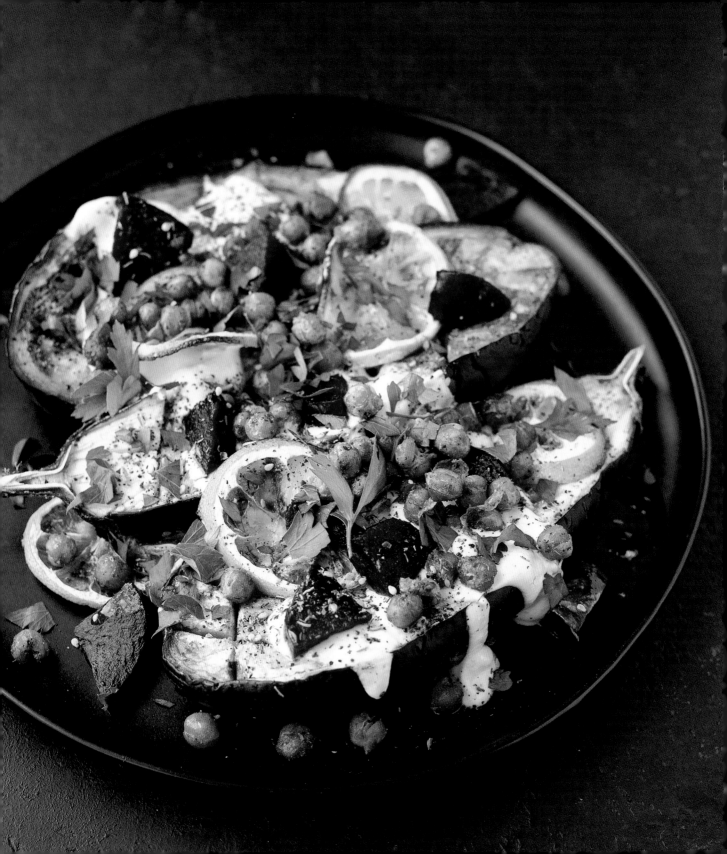

DECONSTRUCTED BABA GANOUSH

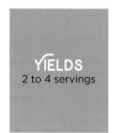

YIELDS
2 to 4 servings

This is one of my favorite recipes from my blog, and I knew I had to share it in my Mediterranean cookbook. Baba ganoush was a regular treat growing up, and I still have fond memories of my Syrian upstairs neighbor pounding, by hand, the charred eggplant. When mom and I heard the pounding, we knew what was up, and she had me run upstairs to get some of my neighbor's memorable baba ganoush.

I took all those smoky and simple flavors and broke them up a bit for this roasted eggplant version. All the flavors of baba ganoush are simplified into a gorgeous and hearty vegetarian meal.

EGGPLANT

1 large eggplant, cut into quarters lengthwise or 2 medium cut in half

3 tbsp (45 ml) olive oil

½ tsp ground cumin

½ tsp ground coriander

¼ tsp salt

1 lemon, sliced thinly

ROASTED CHICKPEAS

1 cup (164 g) cooked or canned chickpeas, drained and rinsed

½ tsp ground cumin

½ tsp paprika

½ tsp za'atar

¼ tsp salt

Ground pepper

2 tbsp (30 ml) olive oil

TAHINI SAUCE

¼ cup (60 ml) tahini

¼ cup (60 ml) 2% or full-fat Greek yogurt

Juice of ½ lemon

1 garlic clove, grated

½ tsp paprika

¼ tsp ground coriander

¼ tsp ground cumin

Pinch of cayenne

¼ tsp salt

Ground pepper

2 tbsp (30 ml) water, to thin out if needed

ADDITIONAL TOPPINGS

Roasted beets, chopped

Fresh parsley, chopped finely

Olive oil, for garnish

Additional za'atar and sea salt

Preheat the oven to 400°F (204°C) and place the cut eggplant in a 9 × 13-inch (22 × 33-cm) baking dish. Use a knife to cut diagonal slits into the flesh but not through the skin and brush oil onto the eggplant.

Season the eggplant with cumin, coriander and salt and top with lemon slices and bake for about 40 minutes. The eggplant should be tender and slightly charred on the outside.

On a baking sheet, toss together the chickpeas, cumin, paprika, za'atar, salt, pepper and oil and roast the chickpeas at the same temperature for about 20 minutes. Once done, remove from the oven and set aside.

Make the tahini sauce in a food processor. Add the tahini, yogurt, lemon juice, garlic, paprika, coriander, cumin, cayenne, salt and pepper and pulse together until smooth. Add water to help thin the sauce—it should be thin enough to spoon over the eggplant, almost a honey-like consistency.

To assemble, spoon the tahini sauce over the eggplant and top with roasted chickpeas. Garnish with beets, parsley, another drizzle of olive oil and a sprinkle of za'atar and sea salt.

TIP: Roasted beets are optional, but you can add them at the same time as you're roasting the eggplant. Just cut them in half, wrap in foil and roast at 400°F (204°C) for about 45 minutes or until tender.

ROASTED TURMERIC POTATOES
WITH MINT FENNEL SLAW

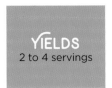

YIELDS
2 to 4 servings

A personal play on the popular Greek-style roasted lemon potatoes, this version is generously dusted with my favorite spice turmeric, giving it a beautiful golden glow. Don't skip the fresh mint fennel slaw as it pairs beautifully with the warm flavors of the potatoes, giving a fun contrast in temperature and texture. Serve as a side dish alongside Pomegranate-Glazed Lamb Chops (page 61) or Yogurt-Marinated Lamb and Eggplant Kabobs (page 54).

TURMERIC POTATOES

4 Yukon gold potatoes, cut into ½-inch (1.2-cm) wedges

1 lemon, zested and juiced

¼ cup (60 ml) olive oil

3 garlic cloves, chopped finely

1 tsp ground turmeric

1 tbsp (3 g) dried oregano

¼ tsp Aleppo pepper flakes

½ tsp salt

MINT FENNEL SLAW

1 fennel bulb, stem removed and sliced thin using a mandoline

1 cup (25 g) loosely packed mint leaves

2 tbsp (30 ml) olive oil

½ lemon, juiced

¼ tsp salt

2 oz (56 g) shaved Parmesan cheese

Preheat the oven to 400°F (204°C) and toss the potatoes with the lemon zest and juice, oil, garlic, turmeric, oregano, Aleppo pepper and salt and arrange on a foil-lined baking sheet in a single layer.

Roast the potatoes for 25 to 30 minutes until they are golden brown and the edges are slightly charred. Remove from the oven and set aside.

To make the slaw, toss together the fennel, mint, oil and lemon juice and season with salt. Top the warm potatoes with the slaw and Parmesan and serve immediately.

 TIP: This dish can be made at the last minute, but if you do have the time, soak the sliced potatoes in a bowl of cold water for as long as you can. The potatoes will release some starch, making them crispier.

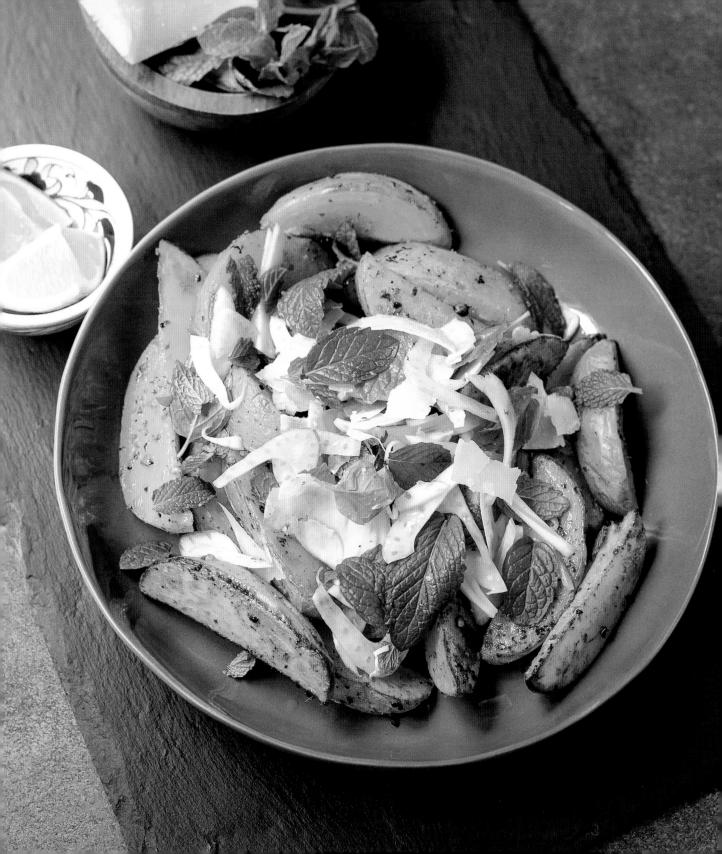

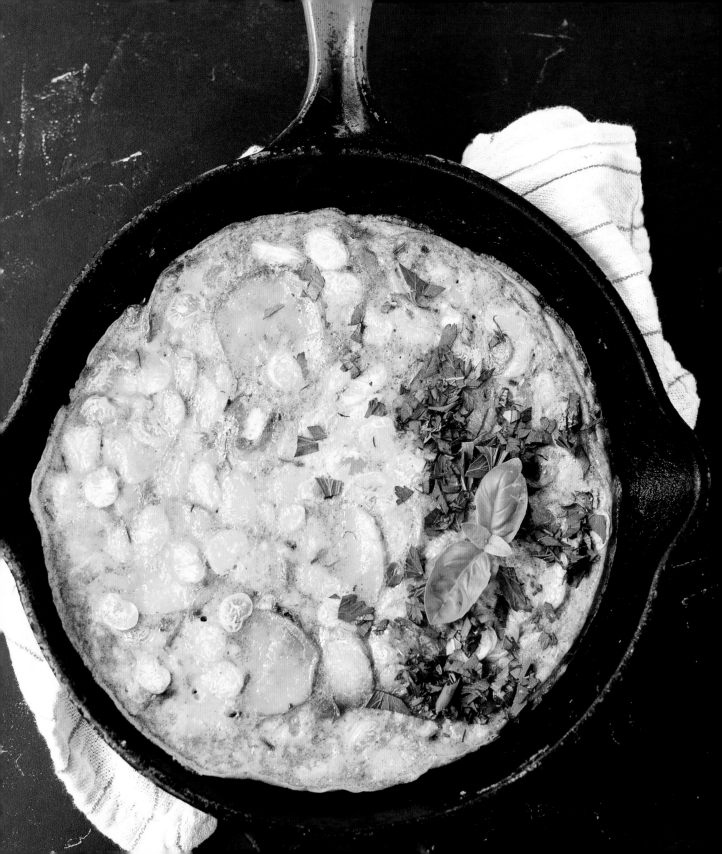

MEDITERRANEAN-STYLE BAKED OMELET WITH POTATOES AND LIMA BEANS

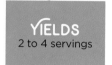

YIELDS
2 to 4 servings

Frittatas is what we normally associate with a baked egg dish, but in Spain they call it a tortilla or Spanish omelet, and it is usually enjoyed in the middle of the day or as a main course at dinner. My very simple and Mediterranean-inspired take on a Spanish tortilla has thin slices of potatoes, earthy turmeric and chewy lima beans. Serve hot or at room temperature and, for an extra bite of saltiness, top with crumbled feta.

2 tbsp (30 ml) olive oil

1 large Yukon gold potato, sliced very thin using a mandoline

4 eggs

1 tsp milk

½ tsp ground turmeric

¼ tsp salt or more as needed

1 cup (178 g) fresh or frozen and thawed lima beans

Chopped mint leaves, for garnish

Heat a 13- to 15-inch (33- to 38-cm) skillet over medium-high heat and add the olive oil and sliced potatoes. Arrange the potatoes in as much of a single layer as possible and cover with a lid, cooking for 5 to 8 minutes or until the potatoes begin to soften and edges begin to crisp up. Flip the potatoes over as needed so both sides get a golden color.

In a bowl, whisk together the eggs, milk, turmeric and salt and reduce the heat to low-medium. Pour the egg mixture into the pan, making sure all the potatoes are evenly coated and scatter the lima beans over the top.

Cover with a lid and continue cooking until the eggs are just set, another 8 to 10 minutes.

Once done, remove from the heat and serve immediately or at room temperature. Garnish with chopped mint leaves.

HARISSA-ROASTED BUTTERNUT SQUASH WITH DATES

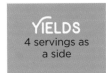

YIELDS
4 servings as a side

Smoky, sweet, spicy and addictive. Cubes of butternut squash are roasted and caramelized along with the spicy harissa sauce. The roasted cubes are tossed with candy-like dates and toasted almonds, and then the creamy tahini is drizzled all over it. This would be a perfect side dish for a holiday party. Sweet potatoes or acorn squash can easily be substituted for the butternut squash.

2–3 lb (907–1360 g) butternut squash, cut into 1-inch (2.5-cm) cubes

2 tbsp (30 ml) olive oil

2 tbsp (30 ml) Easy Homemade Harissa Sauce (page 144)

½ tsp ground sumac

½ tsp garlic powder

¼ tsp ground cinnamon

½ tsp salt

4–5 pitted dates, roughly chopped

¼ cup (23 g) toasted sliced almonds

¼ cup (60 ml) tahini

Chopped parsley, for garnish

Preheat the oven to 400°F (204°C) and line a baking sheet with foil.

Toss together the cubed butternut squash, oil, harissa, sumac, garlic powder, cinnamon and salt and arrange in a single layer on the baking sheet.

Roast the squash for about 40 to 45 minutes, until tender and caramelized on the outside.

Remove the roasted squash from the oven and transfer it to a serving platter. Top with the dates and almonds. Drizzle with the tahini or serve on the side for dipping. Garnish with chopped parsley.

 TIP: Save prep time and buy peeled and cut butternut squash at your local market.

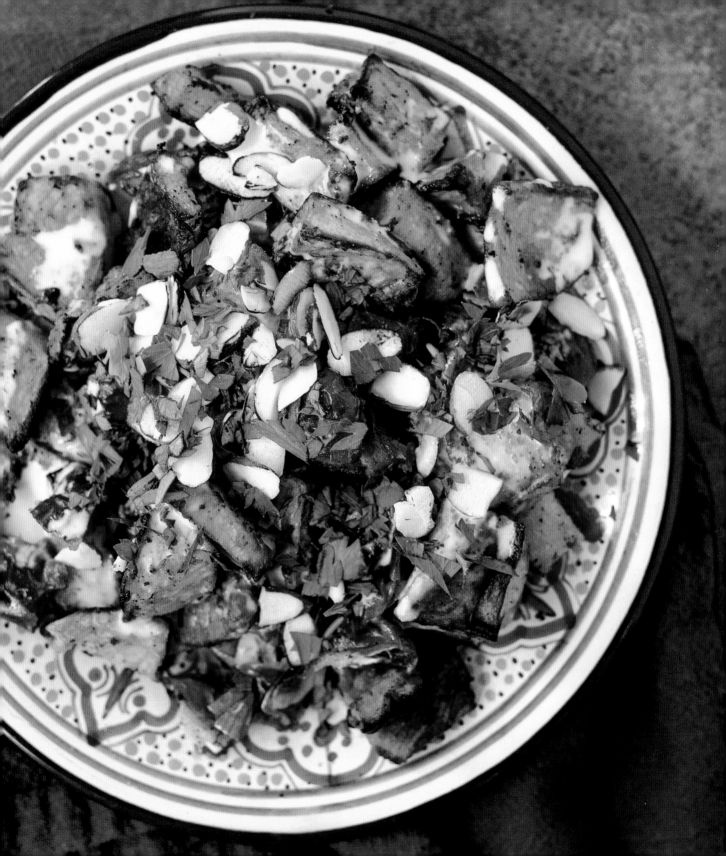

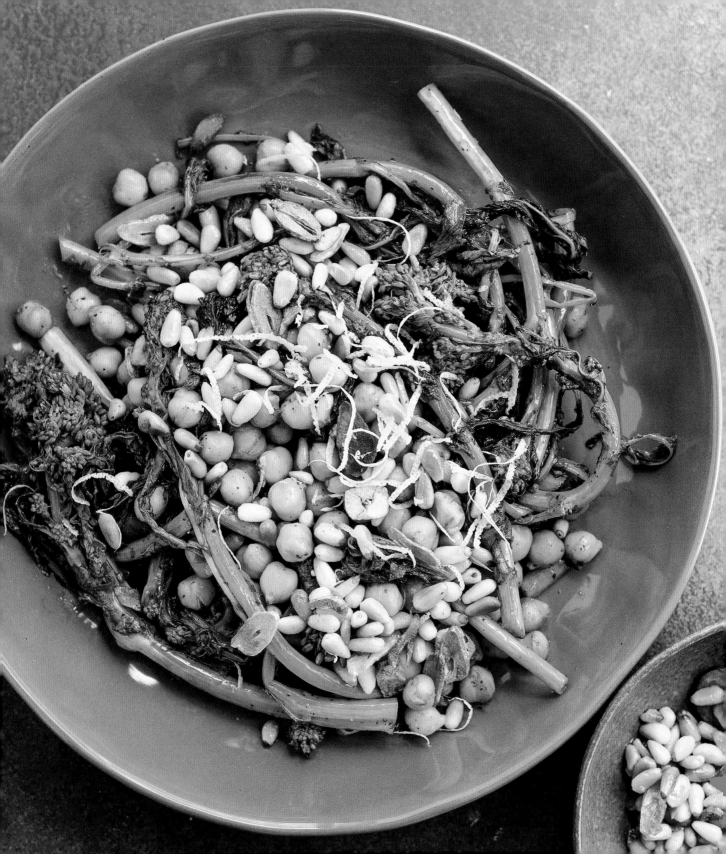

BROCCOLI RABE WITH CHICKPEAS AND GARLIC PINE NUTS

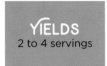

YIELDS
2 to 4 servings

Also called rapini, broccoli rabe is popular in Italian cuisine. It is closely related to the turnip family and has a wonderful bitter, mustardy flavor. In this recipe, I lightened up its mustard flavor with bright lemon zest and garnished it with savory garlic slices and toasted pine nuts. Serve as a side dish alongside Salmon Puttanesca (page 69) or Everyday Chicken Shawarma (page 62).

2 tbsp (30 ml) olive oil

3 garlic cloves, thinly sliced

¼ cup (34 g) pine nuts

1 bunch broccoli rabe

1 cup (164 g) cooked chickpeas

1 tsp ground sumac

½ tsp Aleppo pepper flakes

Salt, as needed

2 oz (56 g) freshly grated Parmesan cheese

Zest of 1 lemon

Drizzle a large skillet with oil and place on medium-high heat. Add the garlic and pine nuts and toast until the garlic is a deep golden color and the pine nuts are lightly toasted. Once done, use a slotted spoon to remove, leaving the excess oil in the pan. Reserve the garlic and pine nuts to a plate on the side.

In the same skillet, add the broccoli rabe to the garlic oil. Cover with a lid for a minute to help soften the thicker stems, and then add the chickpeas and season with sumac, Aleppo pepper and salt. Continue cooking until the leaves are wilted and the stems are tender yet crunchy, about 4 to 5 minutes.

Transfer the broccoli rabe and chickpeas to a serving dish and garnish with the garlic and pine nuts, grated Parmesan and lemon zest. Serve immediately.

 TIP: Broccoli rabe is often sold in large bunches. If you're feeding a family of 3 to 4, cook up the entire bunch (it's a lot!); otherwise use half now and half another time. You can eat the whole vegetable, so don't throw away those thick stems—just chop them up a bit!

CAULIFLOWER RICE PILAF WITH LENTILS, FRIED ONIONS AND BURST TOMATOES

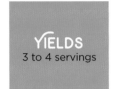

YIELDS
3 to 4 servings

One of my absolute favorite Lebanese dishes is called mujadara, a humble and simple vegetarian rice dish with crispy caramelized onions and brown lentils. Now rice I love, but I have been obsessed with the versatility of riced cauliflower as well, which holds up just as well and absorbs all the warm spices and flavors.

You can make cauliflower rice yourself or use pre-made or frozen riced cauliflower for this recipe.

1 large cauliflower, about 2 lb (907 g), cut into florets

3 tbsp (45 ml) olive oil, divided

1 large sweet or white onion, cut in half and sliced very thinly

½ cup (96 g) dried brown lentils, rinsed

1 tsp ground cumin

½ tsp ground cinnamon

½ tsp ground allspice

½ tsp salt

Ground pepper

8 oz (226 g) cherry tomatoes

¼ cup (6 g) loosely packed mint leaves, roughly chopped

Make the cauliflower rice. Add the florets to a food processor and pulse until you have fine crumbs with a rice-like consistency. One medium-large cauliflower should make about 3 cups (255 g) of riced cauliflower. Set aside.

In a large skillet over medium heat, add 2 tablespoons (30 ml) of oil and the onion. Cook the onion until it softens, reduces in size and becomes a deep golden and slightly charred color, about 10 to 15 minutes. Keep an eye on it so it doesn't burn too quickly. Once done, transfer the onion to a plate and set aside.

As the onion browns, cook the lentils in a medium-size pot with 2 cups (475 ml) of water. Bring the lentils to a boil and then reduce the heat and continue cooking until the lentils are tender but not mushy, about 15 to 20 minutes. Once done, drain and set aside.

Using the same skillet you cooked the onions in, add in the riced cauliflower and season with the cumin, cinnamon, allspice, salt and pepper, Toss to combine and cover the pan with a lid, cooking the cauliflower for 6 to 8 minutes until tender. Stir in the cooked lentils and the caramelized onions.

Add 1 tablespoon (15 ml) of oil to a small skillet and bring to medium-high heat. Add the tomatoes and a pinch of salt and cook the tomatoes until they begin to burst and soften.

Arrange the cauliflower pilaf on a platter and top with the burst cherry tomatoes and garnish with mint.

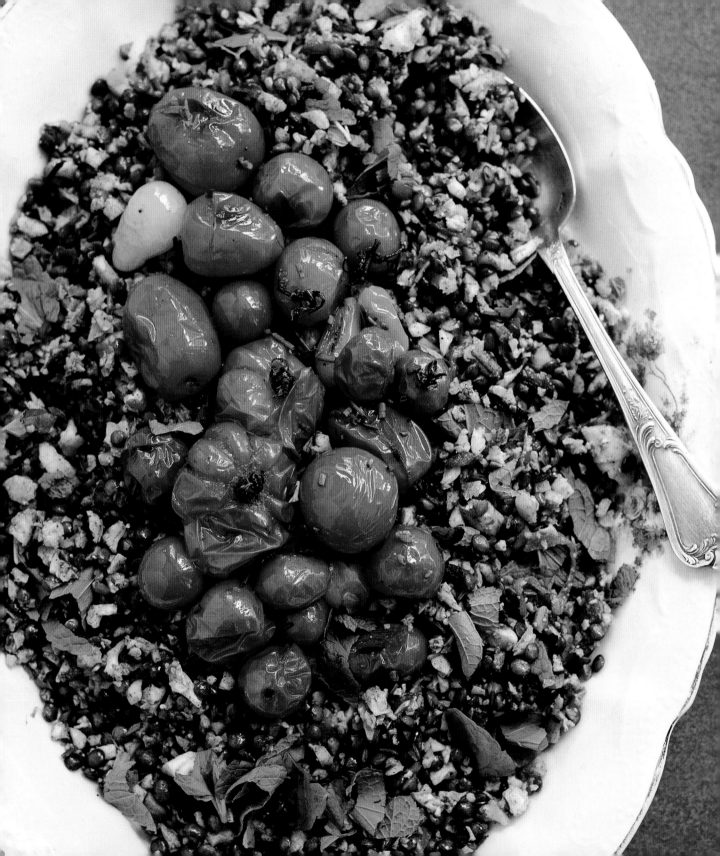

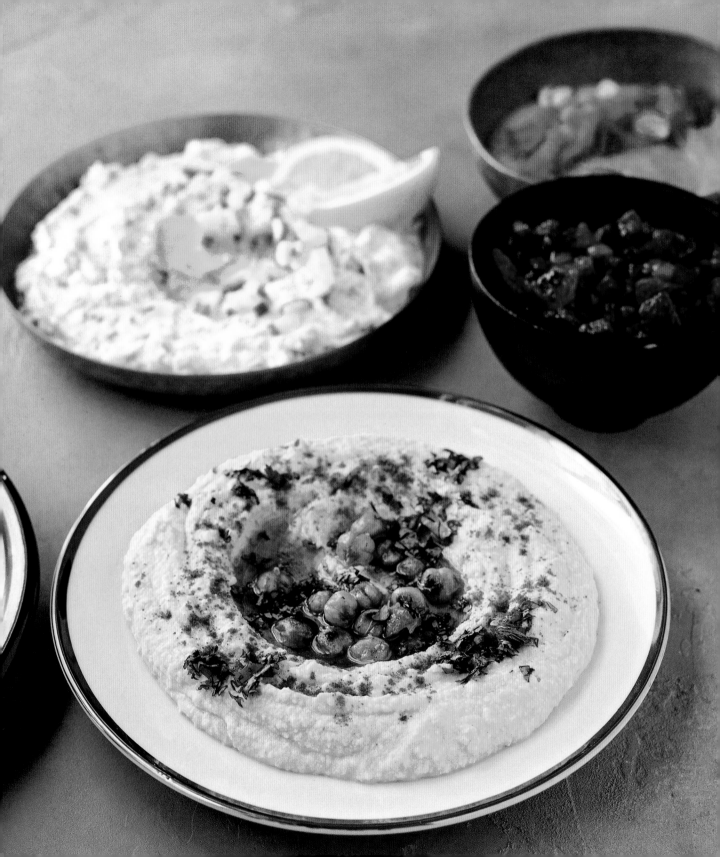

CHAPTER 5

SAUCES, DIPS AND SPREADS

AROMATIC CONDIMENTS TO ENHANCE ANY DISH

This was my absolute favorite chapter to create. Sauces, dips and spreads are so much fun and can be used in a multitude of ways.

Easy Homemade Harissa Sauce (page 144) is used throughout this book. Not only is it fabulous as a condiment with Za'atar Chicken Skewers (page 65), it can also be used to garnish dishes like the Cumin-Scented Squash and Lentil Soup with Crispy Chickpeas (page 81).

Magical Herb Tahini Sauce (page 147) is just that—absolutely magical! You'll want to make an extra batch to slather onto sandwiches or wraps, or to use as a dip for Grilled Za'atar-Spiced Flatbread with Squash Blossoms (page 38) or Red Lentil Falafel (page 111).

Blood Orange and Pomegranate Salsa (page 164) is gorgeous to look at and has layers of sweet, spicy and citrusy flavors. Eat as-is with Spiced Baked Pita Chips (page 42) or as a garnish on top of stuffed eggplant to brighten up the robust flavors.

Have fun with these dips and spreads and use them often. All you need in most cases is a quick whiz of a food processor and you have flavorful condiments ready to add to any dish.

EASY HOMEMADE HARISSA SAUCE

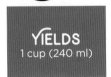

YIELDS
1 cup (240 ml)

This one's for all the spice-lovers out there. Harissa is a fiery chili paste originating in North Africa and gaining in popularity all over the world. There are numerous blends and recipes for harissa, but I like to keep mine simple and smoky. Plop a spoonful on anything you'd like to spice up, such as One-Pot Paprika Chicken with Olives and Orzo (page 49) or on top of hummus for an extra zesty kick.

2 large red bell peppers

3 fresno peppers

4 garlic cloves, peeled

1 tbsp (15 ml) tomato paste

1 tsp ground cumin

1 tsp paprika

1 tsp olive oil, plus more as needed

1 tsp lemon juice

1 tsp lemon zest

Salt, as needed

Preheat the oven to broil or 550°F (287°C) and line a baking sheet with foil. Place the bell peppers and fresno peppers on the baking sheet. Wrap the garlic cloves in a small piece of foil and place on the baking sheet with the peppers. This will ensure that the garlic doesn't burn too quickly.

Broil the peppers and garlic until the entire pepper is softened and you can see black char, about 10 to 12 minutes. Once done, remove the peppers from the oven and cover with another piece of foil and allow to cool enough to handle. This also helps make the outer charred skin easier to remove.

Once cool enough to touch, remove the skin, seeds and stems from the peppers and place the flesh in a food processor along with the roasted garlic cloves.

Add the tomato paste, cumin, paprika, oil and lemon juice and zest to the food processor and pulse until there is a smooth yet coarse consistency. Taste for seasoning and add salt as needed.

Pour the harissa into an airtight container and keep in the fridge for up to 4 days.

 TIP: If fresno peppers aren't in season, use serrano peppers which will provide about the same level of heat but may show small specks of green in the sauce.

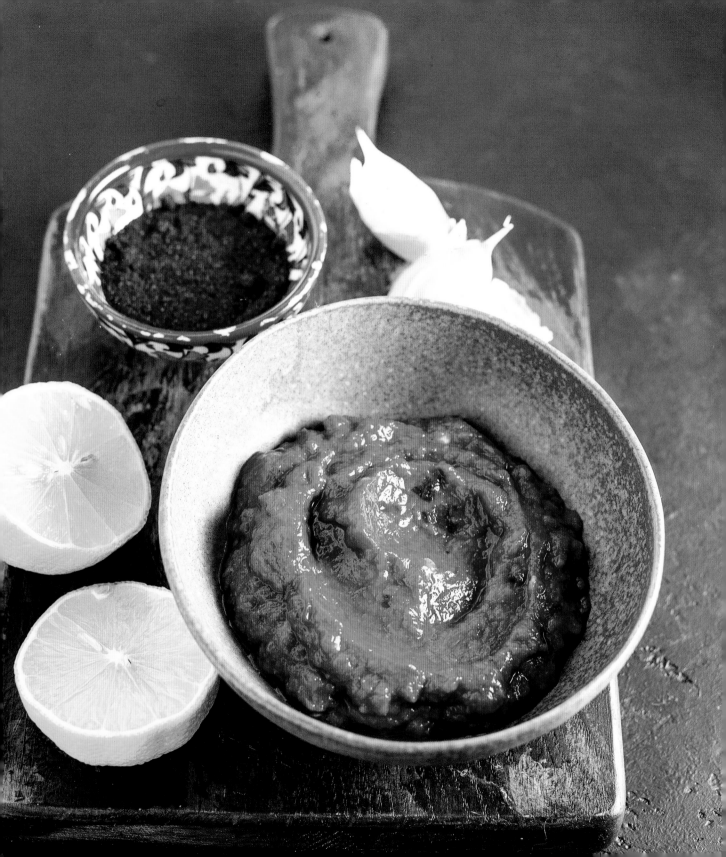

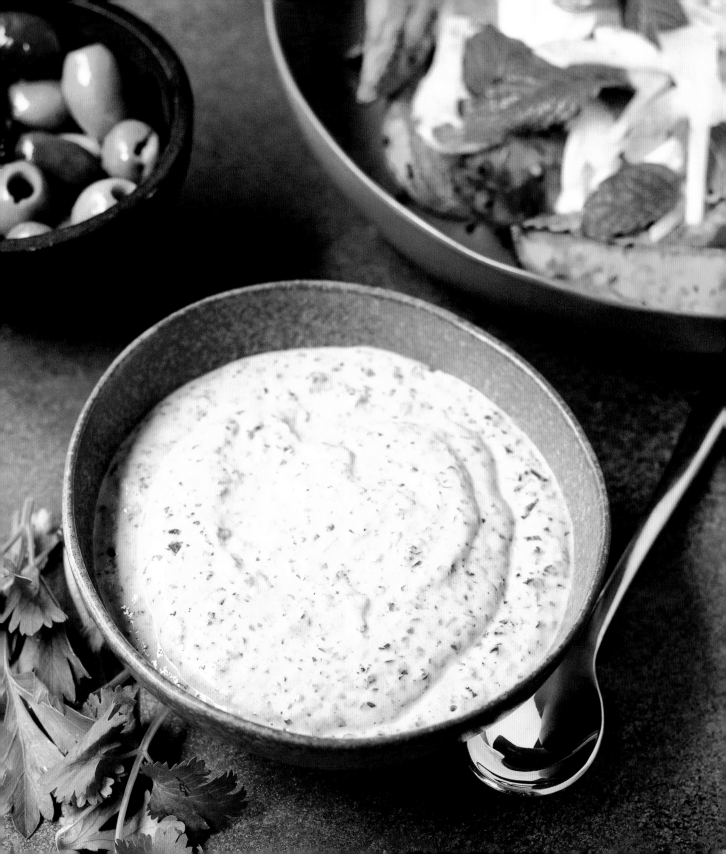

MAGICAL HERB TAHINI SAUCE

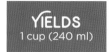

YIELDS
1 cup (240 ml)

This sauce will be your new obsession. It is full of fresh herbs and nutty, creamy tahini and is absolutely delicious with everything you put it on. Slather this green tahini on some toasted bread with fresh tomatoes or serve it alongside Yogurt-Marinated Lamb and Eggplant Kabobs (page 54) or Za'atar Chicken Skewers (page 65).

½ cup tahini

½ cup (10 g) fresh cilantro leaves hard stems removed

½ cup (10 g) fresh parsley leaves, hard stems removed

½ cup (10 g) fresh mint leaves

1 lemon, zested and juiced

2 garlic cloves, roughly chopped

¼ tsp ground cumin

Pinch of cayenne (optional, for heat)

Salt, as needed

½ cup water

1 tbsp (15 ml) olive oil

Place the tahini, cilantro, parsley, mint, lemon zest and juice, garlic, cumin, cayenne, salt, water and oil in a food processor and blend until well incorporated. Use a small spatula to scrape down the sides periodically and taste for seasoning. You're looking for a pourable consistency similar to honey. Add more water if needed for desired texture.

 TIP: This green tahini sauce works with just about any proportion of the listed herbs. The trick is, the herbs must always be fresh. Substitute basil for the cilantro if you aren't a cilantro fan.

PISTACHIO PESTO

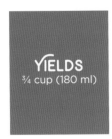

YIELDS
¾ cup (180 ml)

I often make a batch of this pesto and use it for the entire week. A slightly different take on the traditional Italian pesto with pine nuts and basil, this version has a wonderful bright twist. Fresh mint leaves, basil and pistachios are all blended together with the usual accompaniments, creating a chunky and slightly tangy pesto.

This pistachio pesto is fabulous as a dip with Spiced Baked Pita Chips (page 42), or alongside Za'atar Chicken Skewers (page 65) or a large helping of roasted vegetables, such as in the Mediterranean Ratatouille with Pistachio Pesto (page 128). The lemon helps keep this pesto fresh for up to 4 days.

¾ cup (96 g) shelled pistachios

¼ cup (25 g) grated Parmesan cheese

½ cup (120 ml) olive oil, divided

1 lemon, zested and juice

½ cup (10 g) loosely packed basil leaves

½ cup (10 g) loosely packed mint leaves

¼ tsp salt

In a food processor, add the pistachios, cheese, ¼ cup (60 ml) oil, lemon zest and juice, basil, mint and salt and blend until incorporated. Slowly stream in the rest of the olive oil until blended. Use a small spatula to scrape down the sides, making sure there are no large pieces. Taste and adjust the seasoning as desired.

 TIP: This pesto freezes up incredibly well. Freeze in an ice cube tray and once completely frozen, transfer to a resealable plastic bag and use as needed.

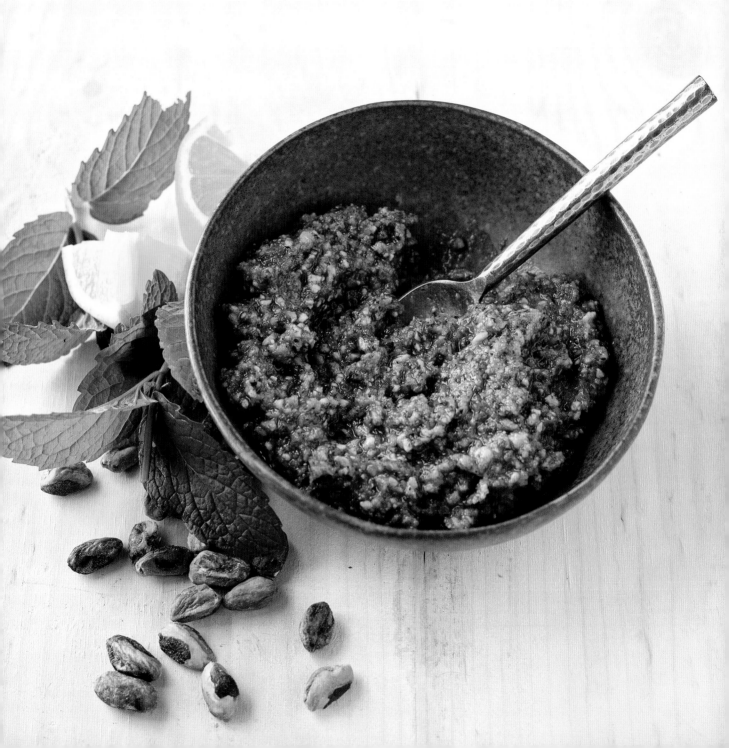

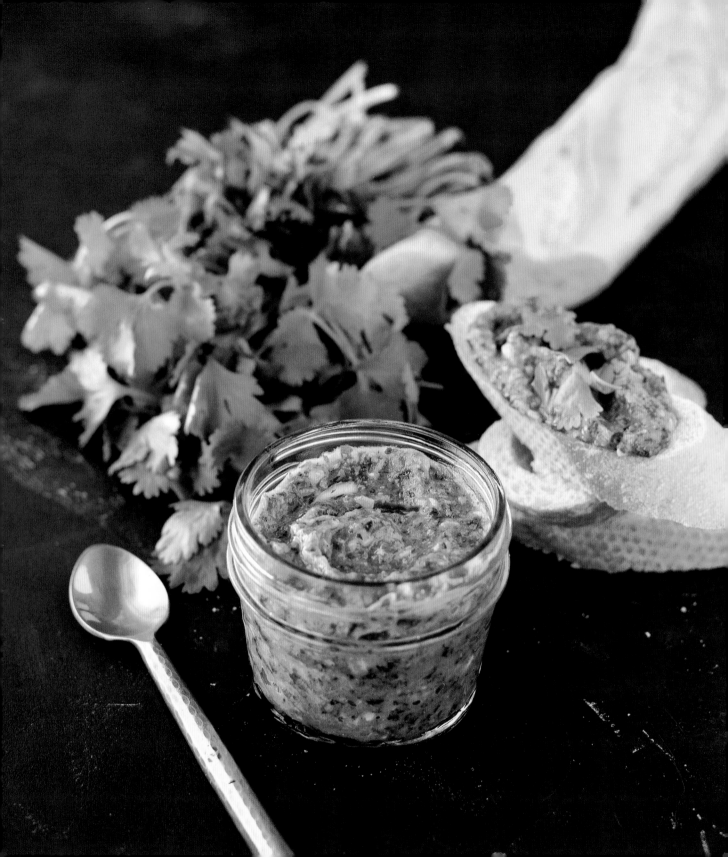

MEDITERRANEAN GREEN ROMESCO

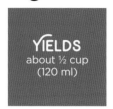

YIELDS
about ½ cup
(120 ml)

I will never forget the first time I had true Spanish romesco—a sauce thickened with nuts and roasted peppers and used to smother anything you'd like. Typically, romesco is made with sweet roasted red peppers, but in my version, I played with different colors and textures to create a green romesco by adding fresh cilantro for brightness.

Serve this as a spread on sandwiches or wraps, with roasted vegetables or just some simply grilled bread. Make a batch, as it keeps in an airtight container for up to 4 days.

1 pasilla pepper

2 Anaheim peppers

1 garlic clove, roughly chopped

4 oz (113 g) slivered or sliced toasted almonds

½ cup (10 g) loosely packed cilantro leaves

¼ cup (60 ml) olive oil

½ tsp paprika

1 tsp red wine vinegar

¼ cup (60 ml) water, as needed for consistency

¼ tsp salt

Preheat the oven to 425°F (218°C) and arrange the peppers on a foil-lined baking sheet. Roast the peppers until the skins are blackened and charred, about 45 minutes.

Remove the roasted peppers from the oven and cover with another piece of foil or plastic wrap and allow to sit for at least 10 minutes. This will help make peeling the charred skins off much easier. Once cool enough to handle, peel and remove the stem and seeds.

In a food processor or blender, combine the peppers, garlic, almonds, cilantro, oil, paprika, vinegar, water and salt together until a coarse paste forms. You may need to add a bit more water for desired consistency.

Place in an airtight container and store for up to 4 days.

ROASTED BEET AND YOGURT DIP TWO WAYS

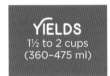

YIELDS
1½ to 2 cups
(360–475 ml)

If I could live off of a vegetable for the rest of my life, it would be beets. Sweet and earthy and gorgeous to look at, I can't help but eat beets in any form that I can think of. This duo of beet dips is a play on one of my favorite soups. Each color has its own flavor element—make one or both and swirl them together. Serve with Spiced Baked Pita Chips (page 42) or your favorite vegetables.

1 lb (453 g) golden beets, scrubbed and stems removed

1 lb (453 g) red beets, scrubbed and stems removed

GOLDEN BEET DIP

⅓ cup (80 ml) 2% or full-fat Greek yogurt

1 tbsp (15 ml) olive oil, plus more for garnish

1 tsp fresh grated ginger

½ tsp ground turmeric

½ lemon, zested and juiced

1 garlic clove, chopped finely or grated

¼ tsp salt, or more to taste

RED BEET DIP

⅓ cup (80 ml) 2% or full-fat Greek yogurt

2 tsp (10 ml) olive oil, plus more for garnish

½ tsp ground cumin

Pinch of cayenne

½ small orange, zested and juiced

¼ tsp salt, or more to taste

Fresh dill, for garnish

Lavash or pita chips, for serving

Preheat the oven to 400°F (204°C) and cut any large beets in half. If they are smaller ones, you can leave them whole.

Wrap the red and yellow beets separately in foil to prevent the colors from bleeding onto each other and roast for about 40 minutes until fork tender.

Allow the roasted beets to cool enough to handle and then peel off the outer layer and roughly chop. Reserve a few chopped roasted beets of each color for the garnish.

For the golden beet dip, add the beets to a food processor along with the yogurt, oil, ginger, turmeric, lemon zest and juice, garlic and salt and pulse until thick and smooth. Taste for seasoning and adjust as needed.

For the red beet dip, add the beets to a food processor along with the yogurt, oil, cumin, cayenne, orange zest and juice and salt and pulse until thick and smooth. Taste for seasoning and adjust as needed.

To serve, layer red and golden beet purees alongside each other and garnish with a drizzle of olive oil, fresh dill and chopped roasted beets. Serve with crispy lavash chips or pita chips.

 TIP: If buying fresh beets with the leaves, don't toss those stems and leaves away! Save them and cook them up as you would any other leafy green, such as spinach or kale.

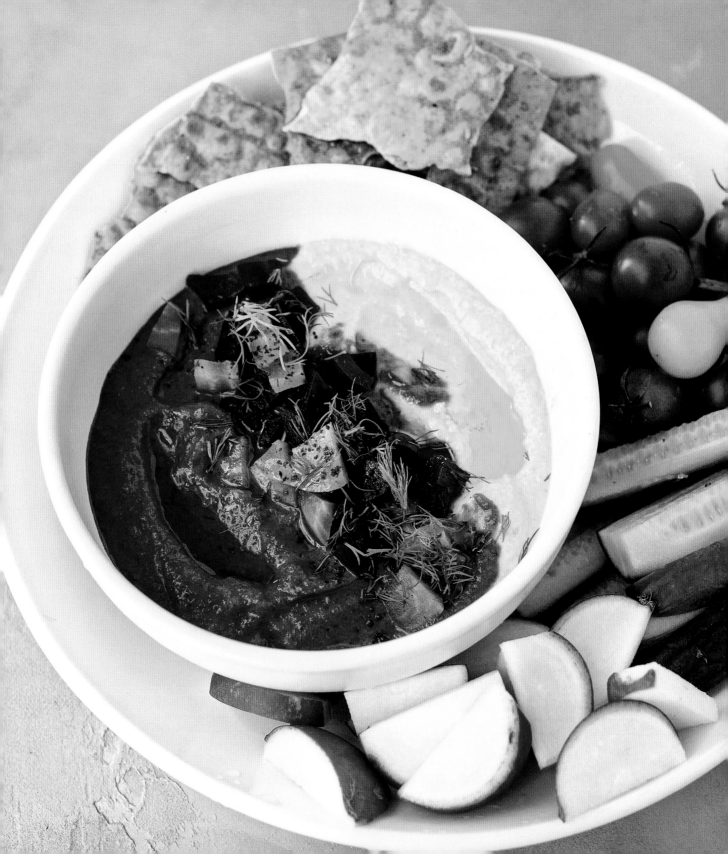

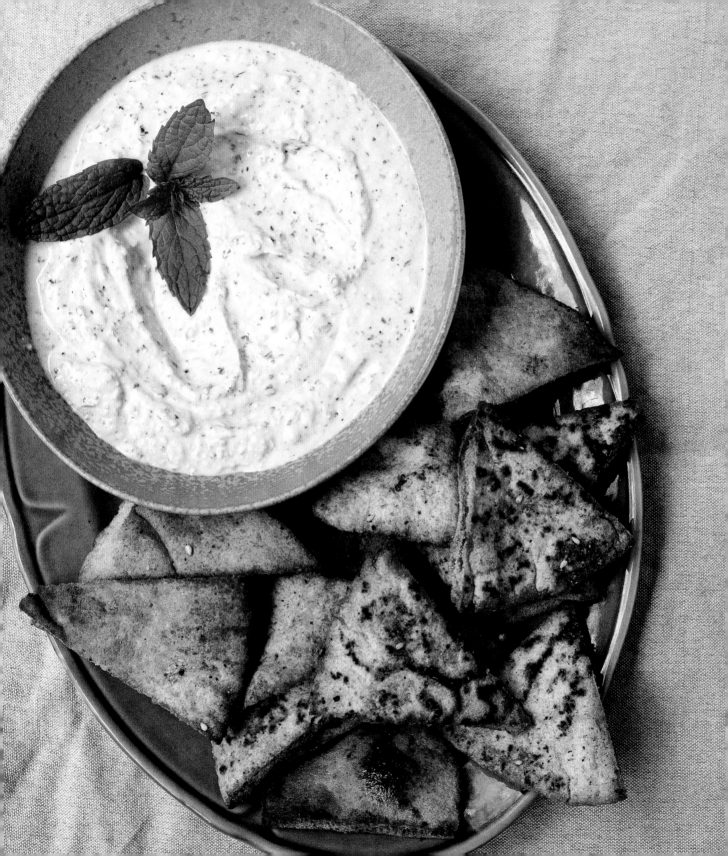

YOGURT FETA DIP WITH FRESH HERBS

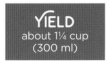

YIELD
about 1¼ cup
(300 ml)

This is one of those dips that makes eating vegetables a bit easier. Creamy and a bit salty, you'll want to dip anything and everything into it.

1 cup (240 ml) plain Greek yogurt

½ cup (75 g) feta cheese

1 lemon, zested and juiced

1 cup (14 g) fresh oregano leaves, stems removed

1 cup (14 g) fresh chives or green onions

1 cup (14 g) fresh parsley leaves, hard stems removed

1 cup (14 g) fresh mint leaves, stems removed

1 garlic clove, roughly chopped

¼ cup (60 ml) olive oil

Salt and pepper, as needed

Add the yogurt, feta, lemon zest and juice, oregano, chives, parsley, mint, garlic and oil to a blender or food processor and blend until combined and smooth. Adjust the seasoning with salt and pepper and serve in a bowl. Garnish with an extra drizzle of olive oil.

PERSIAN STYLE EGGPLANT AND YOGURT DIP

YIELDS
about 1 cup
(240 ml)

Late summer's eggplant is ideal for this dip, which is a true star. Look for eggplants that have a smooth glossy skin and no blemishes or wrinkles. Another tip is to look for smaller, younger eggplants, which won't be as bitter and have fewer seeds.

2 medium eggplant, about 2 lb (907 g)

1 garlic clove, grated

½ lemon, juiced

¼ cup (60 ml) labneh

½ tsp ground turmeric

½ tsp salt, or more as needed

Olive oil, for garnish

Fresh mint leaves, for garnish

Pomegranate seeds, for garnish

Spice Baked Pita Chips (page 42), for serving

Preheat the oven to 425°F (218°C) and line a baking sheet with foil.

Use a fork to poke holes all over the whole eggplant. For a smokier flavor, you can grill the eggplant over a gas or charcoal grill instead. Roast the eggplant for 35 to 40 minutes, until it is charred on the outside and collapses, which will indicate that it is soft on the inside.

Remove from the oven and allow to cool enough to handle. Cut off the stem and cut it in half to expose the flesh. Use a spoon to scoop out the pulp, leaving behind the skin.

Add the eggplant pulp to a food processor along with the garlic, lemon juice, labneh, turmeric and salt. Pulse just a few times to mix everything together but don't overmix, as that will thin out the dip too much. Taste for seasoning and adjust as necessary

Transfer to a bowl and garnish with a drizzle of olive oil, mint and pomegranate. Serve with Spiced Baked Pita Chips (page 42).

TIP: Labneh is a Middle Eastern strained yogurt that is beautifully thick and slightly tangy. Labneh is becoming more available; however, if you can't find it, feel free to substitute thick full-fat Greek yogurt.

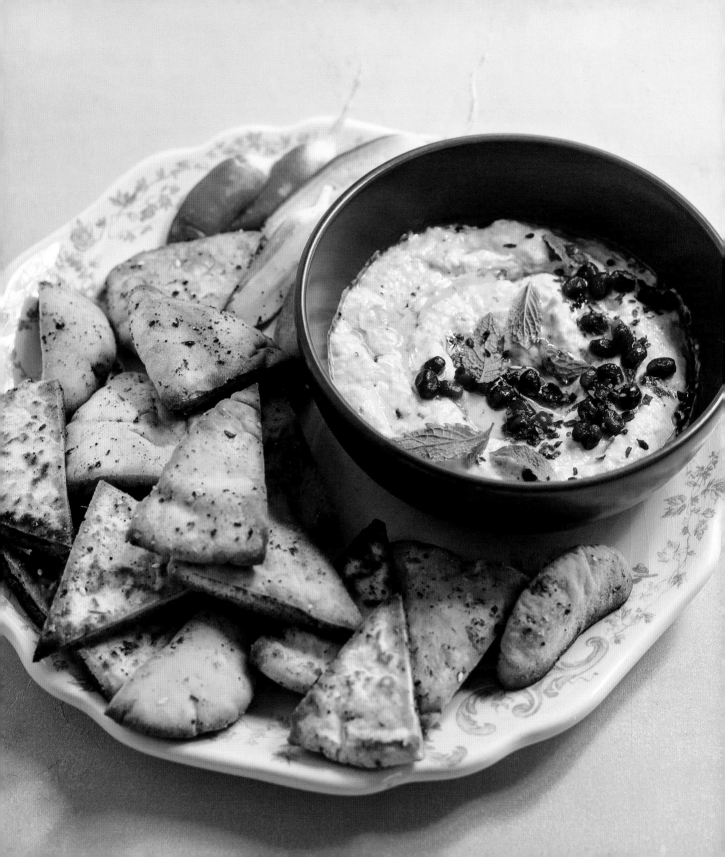

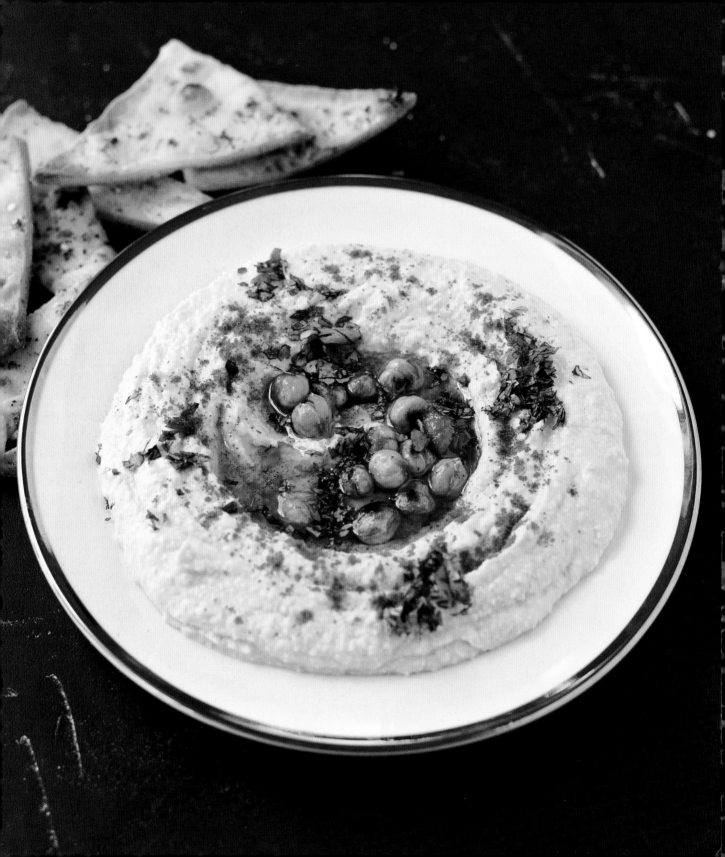

EVERYDAY HUMMUS

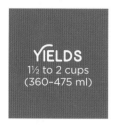

YIELDS
1½ to 2 cups
(360–475 ml)

Hummus purists swear by the traditional and authentic way of making hummus from scratch from dried chickpeas. Delicious, yes, but ultimately time-consuming, since you have to soak the chickpeas overnight before boiling until tender. Good-quality canned chickpeas are an absolute savior when making your own hummus at home. Plus it will be less expensive and healthier than store-bought because you know what you're putting into it. If you insist on making hummus with dried beans, no problem. Soak dried chickpeas overnight and then boil on the stovetop until tender. A pressure cooker speeds up the cooking as well.

2 (15-oz [425-g]) cans chickpeas, liquid reserved

3 tbsp (45 ml) olive oil, plus more for garnish

½ cup (120 ml) tahini

2–3 garlic cloves, chopped finely or grated

¾ tsp ground cumin

¾ tsp salt

½ lemon, juiced

2 tbsp (30 ml) water, plus more if needed

¼ tsp paprika, for garnish

1 tbsp fresh parsley or cilantro, chopped finely for garnish

Spiced roasted chickpeas, for garnish

Open the canned chickpeas and reserve 3 tablespoons (45 ml) of the chickpea liquid (also known as aquafaba) and drain and rinse the rest of the chickpeas. If you have more time, remove the outer skin of the chickpeas and discard.

Add the chickpeas to a food processor along with the oil, tahini, garlic, cumin, salt, lemon juice, aquafaba and water and blend to a smooth consistency. Stop every so often and use a spatula to push down the sides if needed and taste for seasoning. If the hummus is too thick, add a bit more water, a little at a time until the desired consistency is reached.

Transfer the hummus to a plate and use the back of a spoon to make a smooth border around the edge with an indent in the middle. Drizzle with olive oil and sprinkle with the paprika and herbs. Garnish the hummus with spiced roasted chickpeas, such as the ones from the Deconstructed Baba Ganoush recipe on page 131.

Serve at room temperature and place leftovers in an airtight container in the refrigerator for up to 4 days.

TIPS: For an even smoother hummus, take a few extra minutes and remove the outer skin of each chickpea.

Have fun and personalize your hummus with some of your favorite flavors. Some flavor ideas are avocado, roasted bell peppers, olives, roasted garlic or roasted beets.

CUCUMBER, YOGURT AND MINT DIP

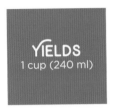

YIELDS
1 cup (240 ml)

I grew up eating this cucumber yogurt dip and would eat spoonfuls of it as I stood in front of the open fridge door. (No judgment if you do the same.) Very similar to the well-known Greek version tzatziki, the Turks call it cacik. We put it on everything and you should, too. A dollop would go deliciously on top of the Unstuffed Grape Leaves (page 107) or with the Meat and Pine Nut Phyllo Rolls (page 18) as well as the Za'atar Chicken Skewers (page 65) or Yogurt-Marinated Lamb and Eggplant Kabobs (page 54). Did I mention it's delicious on everything?

2 medium Persian cucumbers, coarsely shredded

¼ tsp salt or more to taste

1 cup (240 ml) 2% or full-fat Greek yogurt

¼ cup (5 g) loosely packed mint leaves, chopped finely

1 lemon, zested and juiced

1 garlic clove, grated

1 tbsp (15 ml) olive oil, for garnish

Place the cucumber in a colander over a bowl or sink and sprinkle with salt. Lightly toss so the salt coats evenly and allow it to sit for 10 minutes. Squeeze as much moisture out of the cucumbers as you can. This will create a thicker yogurt dip and not leave it watery.

Transfer the cucumber to a bowl along with the yogurt, mint, lemon zest and juice and garlic.

Mix everything together until well combined and taste for seasoning. When ready to serve, garnish with a drizzle of olive oil.

 TIP: Thick Greek yogurt is my personal preference here, but you can easily substitute regular yogurt for a thinner consistency.

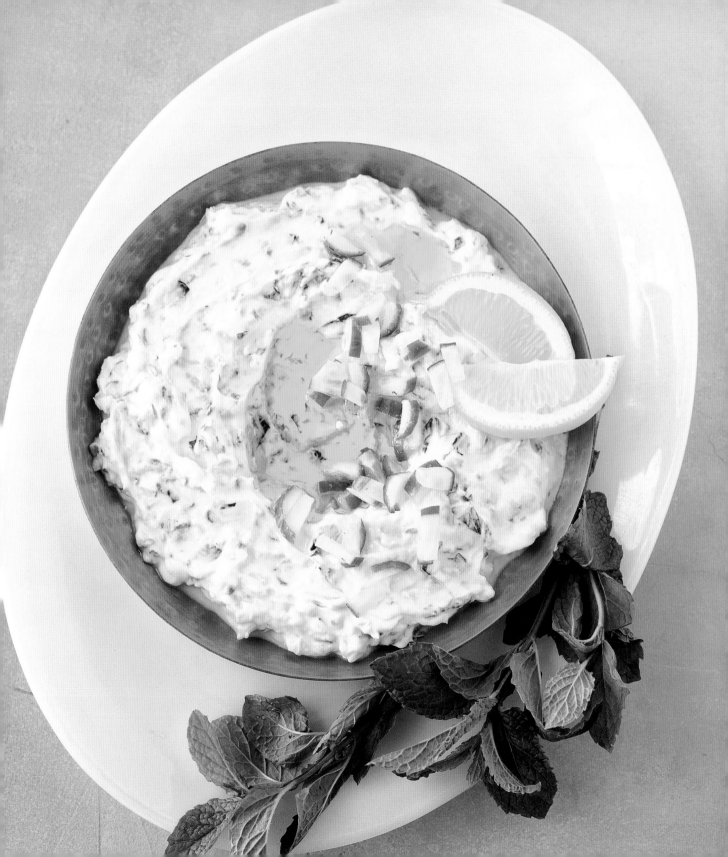

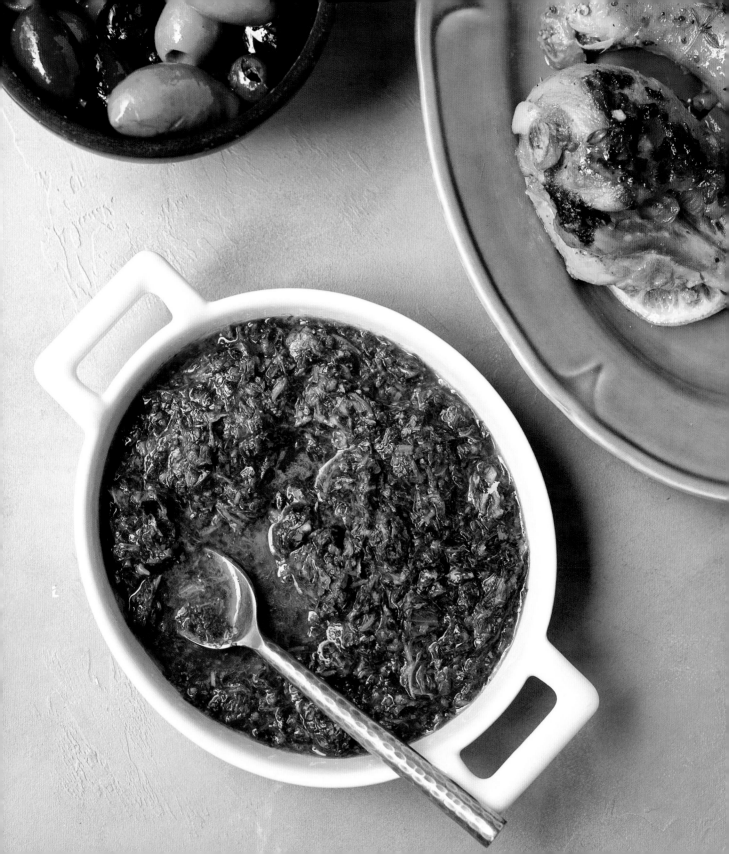

MEDITERRANEAN CHIMICHURRI

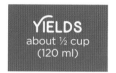

YIELDS
about ½ cup
(120 ml)

The addition of mint brightens up this not-so-traditional chimichurri sauce. A quick blend of fresh herbs with lemon and garlic, this Mediterranean chimichurri lasts for days in the fridge. Spoon over Pomegranate-Glazed Lamb Chops (page 61) or on top of Everyday Hummus (page 159) for a fresh bite. If cilantro isn't your jam, feel free to substitute with all parsley and mint.

2 garlic cloves, roughly chopped

1 lemon, zested and juiced

¾ cup (20 g) loosely packed cilantro, hard stems removed

¾ cup (20 g) loosely packed parsley, hard stems removed

¼ cup (5 g) mint leaves

3 tbsp (45 ml) olive oil

¼ tsp salt

Add the garlic, lemon zest and juice, cilantro, parsley, mint, oil and salt to a food processor and pulse to blend. Continue pulsing until the mixture is almost as thick as pesto, has a deep bright green color and has no large garlic pieces or oversized leaves left.

BLOOD ORANGE AND POMEGRANATE SALSA

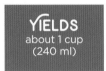

YIELDS
about 1 cup
(240 ml)

This salsa is a play on some of my favorite Turkish flavor pairings. Blood oranges are tart and have a gorgeous color and pair beautifully with the deep red pomegranate jewels. Because this salsa has a wonderful tart spicy flavor, I'd suggest spooning it over Stuffed Eggplant with Meat and Tahini (page 58) or serving as a side with Spiced Baked Pita Chips (page 42).

3 medium blood oranges, peeled, seeded and chopped into ¼-inch (6-mm) pieces

⅔ cup (150 g) pomegranate seeds

1 cup (170 g) peeled and chopped roasted beets, cut into ¼-inch (6-mm) pieces

1 small serrano or fresno pepper, seeded and chopped finely

1 garlic clove, chopped finely

1 tsp honey

1 tsp olive oil

⅓ cup (10 g) fresh cilantro, stems removed and chopped

¼ tsp salt, or as needed

Add the oranges, pomegranate, beets, pepper, garlic, honey, oil, cilantro and salt to a bowl and stir to combine. Place in airtight container in the fridge for up to 4 days.

TIP: If blood oranges aren't in season, feel free to substitute navel or cara cara oranges. It will be a bit more sweet overall, but it will still have a beautiful balance of flavors.

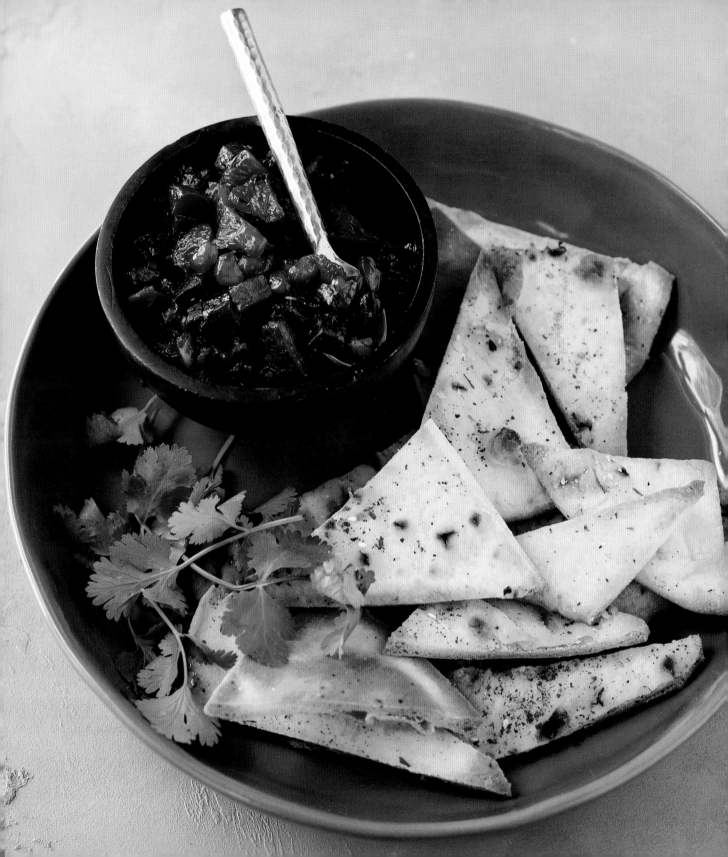

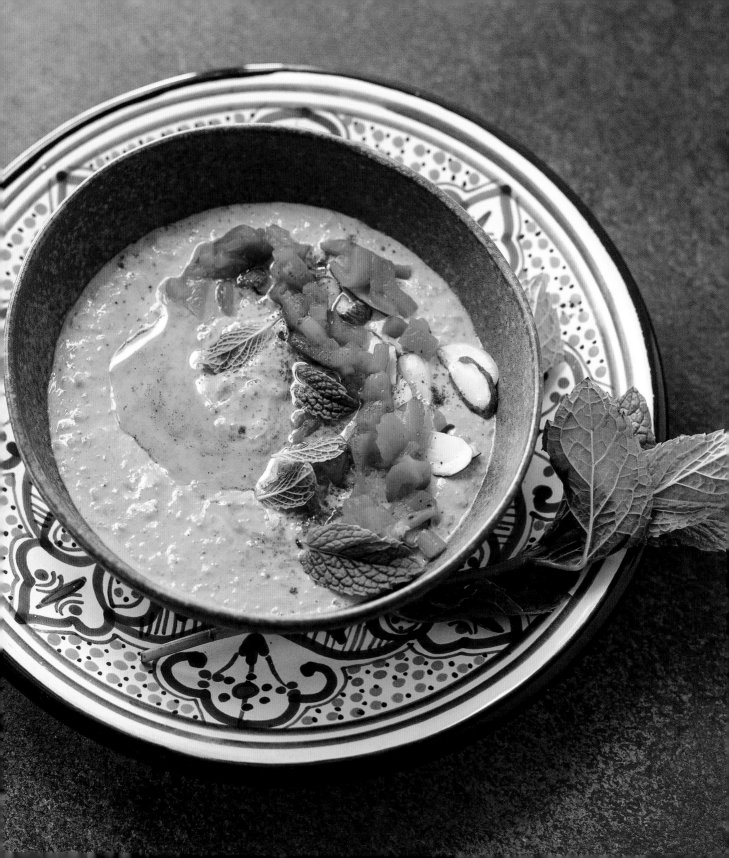

ROASTED RED PEPPER AND TAHINI SPREAD

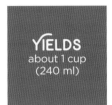

YIELDS
about 1 cup
(240 ml)

The first time I had roasted red pepper dip I was sitting off the sidewalk in Istanbul. I had never tasted anything like it before. It was sweet, smoky and smooth, and I couldn't wait to recreate a similar dish when I got home. Traditionally made with walnuts and roasted peppers, the Turkish spread is called muhammara. Instead, I gave it a smoother twist by adding creamy tahini and toasted almonds and smoked paprika for a warm kick.

Drizzle some over Red Lentil Falafel (page 111) before wrapping it all up in a pita.

2 whole roasted peppers, roughly chopped, divided

¼ cup (23 g) toasted sliced almonds, divided

3 garlic cloves, roughly chopped

½ tsp ground cumin

½ tsp smoked paprika

Pinch of cayenne

¼ tsp salt

½ lemon, juiced

½ cup (120 ml) tahini

2 tbsp (30 ml) olive oil, plus more for garnish

2 tbsp (30 ml) water, if needed for consistency

Reserve some pepper and almonds for the garnish. In a food processor, add the peppers, almonds, garlic, cumin, paprika, cayenne, salt, lemon juice, tahini and oil and blend until smooth. If the spread is too thick, drizzle in a little bit of water at a time and blend until the desired consistency is reached.

Transfer to a bowl and garnish with peppers, almonds and a drizzle of olive oil.

TIP: Tahini is a nutty-flavored sesame seed paste that is perfect for creamy dips, sauces and dressings, especially if you or someone you know has a nut allergy. You can often find tahini in the peanut butter aisle of your local store. Use a spoon to mix it up a bit as the oil will float to the top.

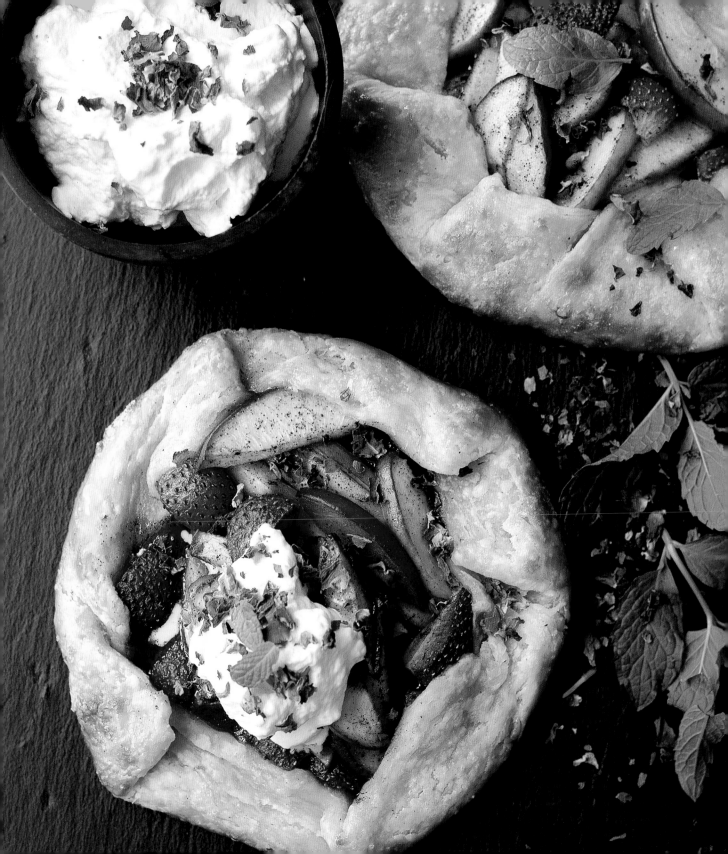

CHAPTER 6

SWEETS AND SIPS

LIGHT AND FRUITY TREATS TO SATISFY YOUR SWEET TOOTH

"I just need one bite," is often what I say after dinner to curb my determined sweet tooth.

Sweets are an integral part of Turkish and Middle Eastern cuisine. Flavors of floral rose water and orange blossom perfume Mediterranean treats ever-so-gently with an exotic and alluring background note. A little rose water goes a mighty long way. If used with a heavy hand, it can make a light fruit flavor quickly turn into a soapy mess.

My favorite dessert in this book, Fruit Rose Tart with Rose Whipped Cream (page 174), is worth baking on a weekday. The combination of seasonal fruit with a touch of rose water brings out the fruit's natural sweetness with a gorgeous light feel. Everything from strawberries, raspberries and plum fruits pairs beautifully with rose water, so use what's in season or what's available to you.

Mini Baklava Bites (page 173) are quick and easy to prepare and take only half the time as traditional baklava. Instead of layering each phyllo sheet one by one, ready-made petite phyllo cups can hold the nut mixture perfectly and can also handle being soaked in the luxurious syrup.

Tahini is a favorite in savory dishes, but it is versatile and creamy enough for desserts as well. Tahini Date Bites with Cardamom (page 182) are a perfect sweet treat or snack with almost a truffle feel.

And because we made it through the weekday with our heads held high, cocktails are in order! Let me tell you, there is nothing more thirst-quenching than a refreshing Muddled Mint and Cucumber Cooler (page 186) on a warm summer's day.

BAKED CARDAMOM FRENCH TOAST WITH PEACHES AND ORANGE BLOSSOM

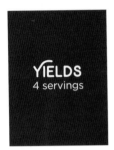

YIELDS
4 servings

Notably, I am a savory breakfast partaker. However, the gentle whiff of orange blossom in a dreamy and easy French toast bake has me excited in every way possible. I have been known to enjoy baked French toast as dessert, too.

Instead of standing in front of the stove griddling one French toast serving at a time, my baked-all-in-one-pan version makes it incredibly easy on any day of the week.

If peaches aren't in season, both raspberries and strawberries pair beautifully with the orange blossom syrup. In addition to breakfast, serve baked cardamom French toast as part of your after dinner dessert with a scoop of thick Greek yogurt and drizzle of peach syrup.

FRENCH TOAST

8–10 slices brioche, cut into ½-inch (1.2-cm) slices

3 whole eggs

2 egg whites

¾ cup (180 ml) whole milk

1 tsp ground cardamom

1 tsp vanilla extract or vanilla paste

2 tbsp (30 g) brown sugar

1 small orange, zest and juice

¼ cup (35 g) chopped pistachios, for garnish

PEACH SYRUP

1 large peach, pit removed and sliced thin

1 tbsp (15 ml) honey

¼ cup (60 ml) water

2 tbsp (30 ml) maple syrup

Pinch of salt

1 tbsp (15 ml) lemon juice

1 tsp orange blossom water

Preheat the oven to 350°F (176°C).

Overlap the brioche slices in a 7 × 10-inch (18 × 25-cm) oven-safe baking dish and set aside.

In a large bowl, whisk together the eggs and egg whites, milk, cardamom, vanilla, brown sugar and orange zest and juice and pour over the brioche. It's OK if some of the bread is sticking out; it does not have to be fully submerged.

Bake the brioche for 25 minutes until you can stick a knife in the center and it comes out clean.

While the toast is baking, make the peach syrup. In a small pot, add the sliced peaches, honey, water, maple syrup and a pinch of salt. Bring to medium heat and allow the peaches to poach in the liquid, until slightly thickened, about 10 minutes.

When it reaches the consistency of natural maple syrup, turn off the heat and stir in the lemon juice and orange blossom water.

Once the French toast is done, remove from the oven and allow it to cool for 5 minutes. Pour the peaches and syrup over the top. Garnish with pistachios.

TIP: Save the egg yolks and use them in the Lemony Chicken Soup with Rice (page 78).

If brioche isn't available, challah bread would be a delicious substitute.

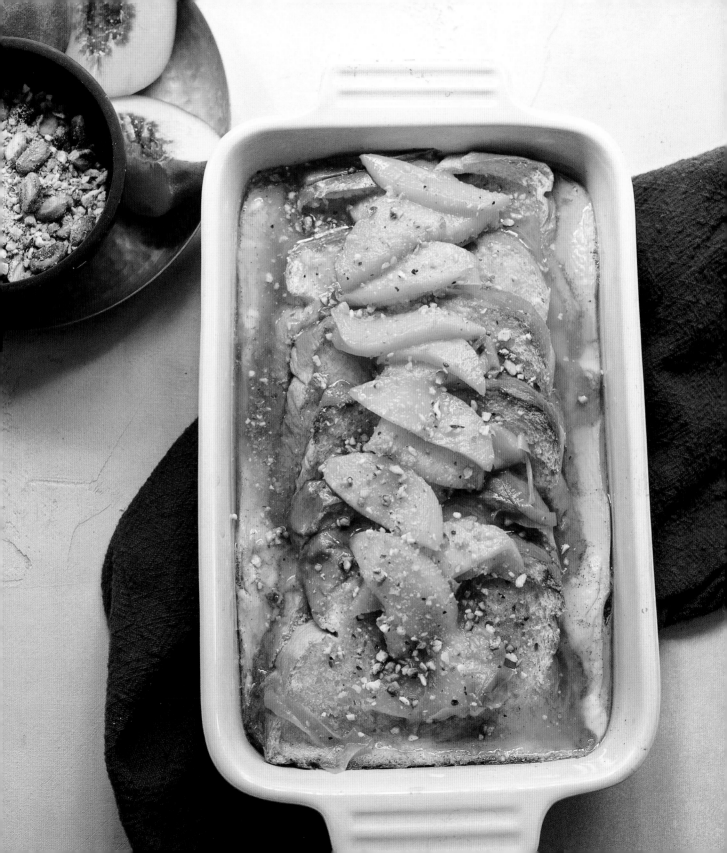

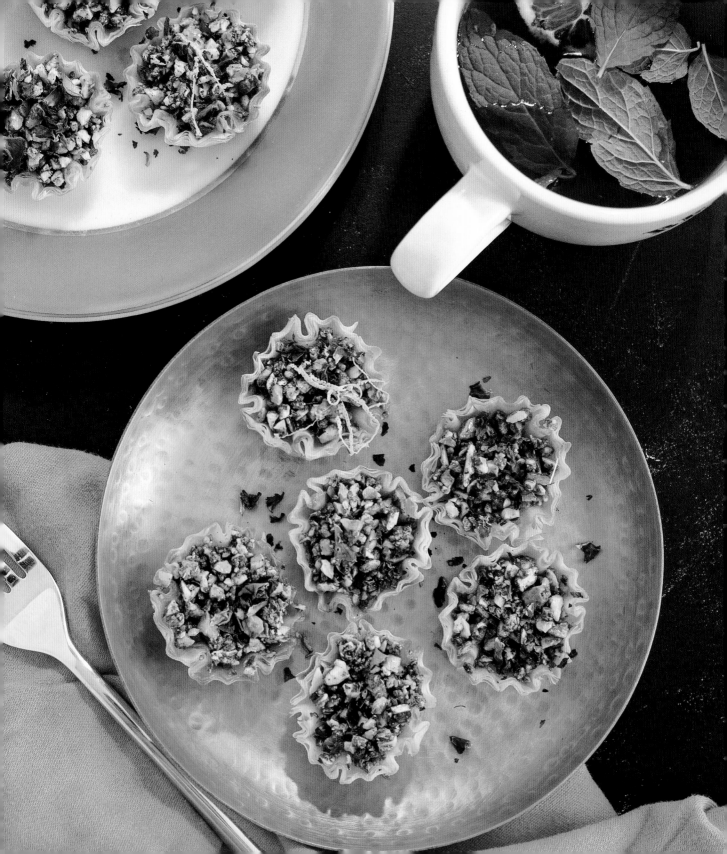

MINI BAKLAVA BITES

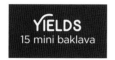
YIELDS
15 mini baklava

Baklava is one of my favorite treats, and it wasn't until we visited Istanbul a few years ago that we really discovered what true baklava is and how to eat it properly. Locals say they know how to spot a tourist by the way they eat their baklava, so stick a fork in it (literally) and you'll be enjoying it just as the Turks do.

MINI BAKLAVA

½ cup (72 g) unsalted almonds

½ cup (62 g) unsalted, shelled pistachios

1 tsp vanilla extract or vanilla paste

1 tsp ground cinnamon

½ tsp ground cardamom

½ tsp ground allspice

Zest of ½ lemon

1 package frozen mini phyllo shells, about 15 to a box

ROSE WATER SYRUP

1 cup (200 g) sugar

½ cup (120 ml) water

1 cinnamon stick

3 strips lemon peel, using a vegetable peeler

2 tsp (10 ml) honey

2 tsp (10 ml) rose water

Preheat the oven to 350°F (176°C).

In a food processor, combine the almonds, pistachios, vanilla, cinnamon, cardamom, allspice and lemon zest and pulse until a fine crumbly consistency with no large nut pieces.

Place the mini phyllo shells on a baking sheet and spoon the nut mixture into the phyllo cups. The nut mixture should come to the top of the cups. Bake for about 10 to 12 minutes.

While the baklava is baking, make the syrup. In a small pot, stir together the sugar and water and add in the cinnamon, lemon peel, honey and rose water. Bring to a gentle boil and cook until the sugar has dissolved and the syrup has thickened slightly, about 5 minutes.

Once the baklava is done, remove from the oven and immediately use a spoon to pour hot syrup over the baklava. Everything should be very hot so the syrup can soak in. You should hear sizzling and see steam as you pour the syrup over.

Allow the baklava to sit for at least 10 minutes so the syrup has a chance to soak in.

Store the baklava in an airtight container at room temperature—the longer it sits, the better it will taste.

TIPS: Mini phyllo shells require a fraction of the work and are easily found in your grocer's frozen section. I suggest keeping an extra box on-hand for quick desserts like this.

If rose water isn't easily sourced, feel free to omit it. You can add a teaspoon of vanilla extract or orange juice to the syrup instead for added essence.

FRUIT ROSE TART
with ROSE WHIPPED CREAM

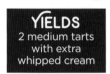

YIELDS
2 medium tarts
with extra
whipped cream

The dough for this tart is a dream to make, and because of the creamy Greek yogurt, the crust is incredibly luxurious without the worry of crumbling. Have fun with the filling and use whatever fruit is in season, such as plums or fresh figs.

DOUGH

1¼ cups (156 g) all-purpose flour, plus more for rolling

8 tbsp (114 g) cold butter, cut into small pieces

2 tbsp (24 g) sugar

¼ teaspoon salt

¼ cup (60 ml) full-fat Greek yogurt

½ lemon, zested and juiced

¼ cup (30 ml) ice cold water

FRUIT FILLING

2 nectarines or peaches, pitted and cut into ¼-inch (6 mm) slices

8 oz (226 g) strawberries, stems removed and cut into quarters

¼ cup (50 g) sugar, plus 1 tbsp (12 g) for garnish

1 tsp vanilla extract or vanilla paste

¾ tsp rose water

Zest of ½ lemon

¼ cup (60 ml) raspberry or strawberry jam

1 egg, beaten

Dried rose petals, for garnish

Mint leaves, for garnish

ROSE WHIPPED CREAM

1 cup (240 ml) whipping cream

1 tbsp (12 g) sugar

½ tsp rose water

Make the dough by adding the flour, butter, sugar and salt into a food processor and pulsing until crumbly.

Whisk together the Greek yogurt, lemon zest and juice and cold water in a bowl and pour the liquid mixture into the food processor. Pulse a few more times until the dough forms. You should be able to squeeze a piece between your fingers, and if it sticks together easily, it's ready.

Lay a large piece of plastic wrap on the counter. Using floured hands, shape the dough into a large disk and wrap it in the plastic. Place the dough in the refrigerator while you prepare the rest of the ingredients.

Preheat the oven to 400°F (204°C) and line a baking sheet with parchment paper.

In another bowl, add together the nectarines and strawberries, ¼ cup (50 g) sugar, vanilla extract, rose water and lemon zest and stir to combine.

Remove the dough from the refrigerator and cut into 2 equal portions. Use a floured rolling pin to roll out the dough into two 10- to 12-inch (25- to 30-cm) circles. At this point, transfer the dough to a baking sheet before filling with fruit.

Spread the jam in the middle of the dough, leaving a 1-inch (2.5-cm) border. Drain any excess liquid from the fruit mixture and divide between the two tarts. Make a small mound of fruit in the middle and fold up the edge of the dough into an overlapping crust.

Brush egg over the exposed dough on both tarts and sprinkle the edges with 1 tablespoon (12 g) of sugar. Bake the tarts for 25 to 28 minutes until the crust is puffed and lightly golden.

Remove from the oven and garnish with dried rose petals and fresh mint.

To make the whipped cream, add the whipping cream, sugar and rose water to a mixing bowl and whisk until aerated and soft peaks form.

Serve the tarts with a dollop of rose whipped cream.

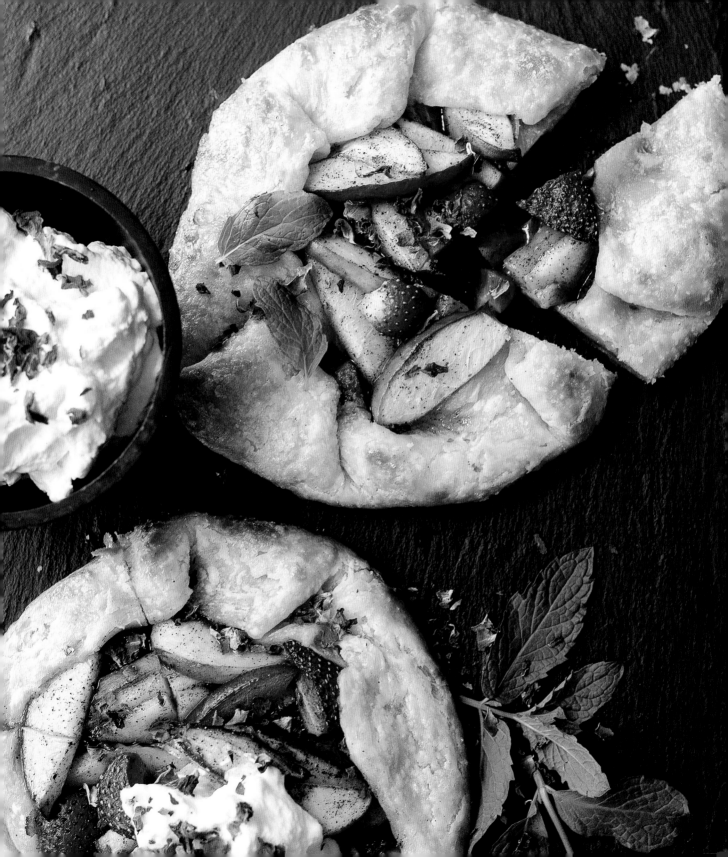

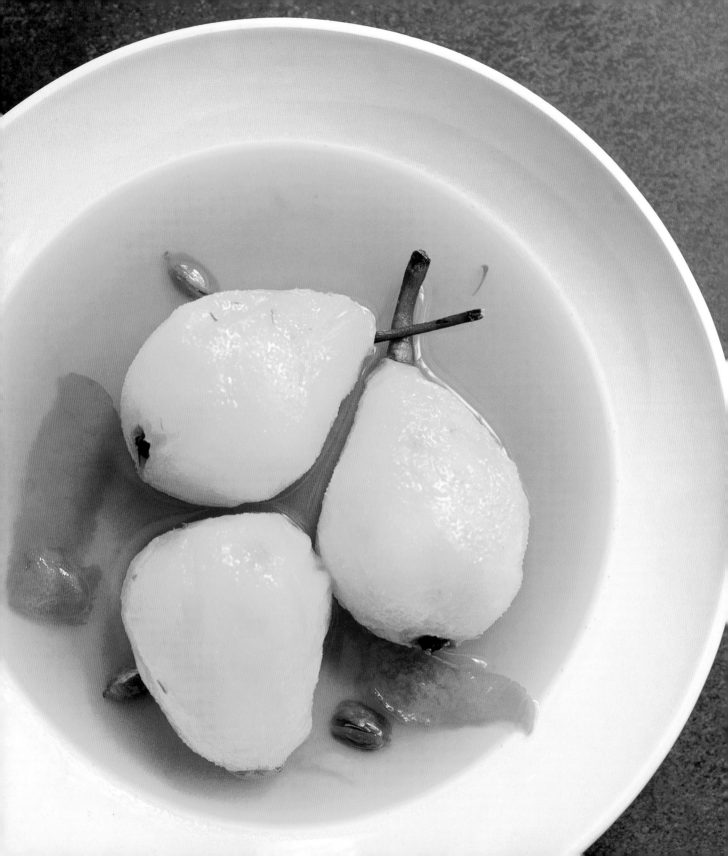

SAFFRON-POACHED PEARS WITH CARDAMOM PODS

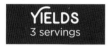
YIELDS
3 servings

Poached pears are one of my favorite sweet treats. As the fruit poaches in the lovely aromatic broth, the liquid reduces, leaving behind a beautiful floral syrup, perfect for pouring over the pears.

¼ tsp saffron threads, crushed

3 whole peeled pears, with stems intact

6 cardamom pods, gently smashed

1 cinnamon stick

4 strips orange zest using a vegetable peeler

1½ cups (360 ml) water

¾ cup (180 ml) white wine

⅓ cup (66 g) sugar

1 tbsp (15 ml) honey

Rose petals, for garnish (optional)

In a medium pot, add the saffron, pears, cardamom, cinnamon, orange zest, water, wine, sugar and honey and bring to a gentle boil. You may need to add a bit more liquid, either water or wine, so the pears are submerged.

Cover the pot and cook the pears on low-medium heat until fork tender, about 20 minutes.

Once done, remove the pears to a bowl and increase the heat to high, reducing the syrup for another 10 minutes. It should be the consistency of light syrup.

Remove the cardamom pods and cinnamon stick and pour the syrup over the pears.

Garnish with rose petals before serving.

TIPS: Save any unused syrup for drinks and cocktails.

Use a mortar and pestle to crush the saffron threads into a powder. This helps intensify its flavor in the syrup.

MINI FIG TARTS WITH POMEGRANATE MOLASSES

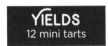

YIELDS
12 mini tarts

When you need a quick and incredibly easy treat, these mini fig tarts satisfy that craving. Pomegranate molasses is quite tart but pairs beautifully with the sweet figs and honey. If fresh figs aren't in season, substitute wedges of fresh plums or even blackberries.

MINI FIG TARTS

1 sheet puff pastry, thawed and cut into 12 equal squares

½ cup (120 ml) pomegranate molasses

2 tbsp (30 ml) honey

1 tbsp (9 g) ground cardamom

12 fresh figs, cut in half lengthwise

¼ cup (56 g) brown sugar

¼ cup (28 g) ground pistachios

Fresh thyme leaves, stems removed, for garnish

ORANGE BLOSSOM YOGURT

¼ cup (60 ml) full-fat Greek yogurt

1 tsp orange blossom water

1 tsp vanilla extract or vanilla paste

1 tbsp (15 ml) honey

1 tsp orange zest

Preheat the oven to 350°F (176°C) and line a baking sheet with parchment paper.

Unroll the thawed puff pastry and use a rolling pin to roll the pastry out a bit so the dough is a bit thinner. Use a sharp knife to cut out 12 equal squares.

In a small bowl, whisk together the pomegranate molasses, 2 tablespoons (30 ml) honey and cardamom until well-combined and spoon about a teaspoon onto each of the pastry squares.

Top each square with 2 halved figs and sprinkle brown sugar over all the fig tarts.

Place the squares on the baking sheet and bake for about 23 to 25 minutes until the pastry is golden brown and the figs have sunken slightly.

Remove the tarts from the oven and garnish with ground pistachios and thyme.

To make the orange blossom yogurt, simply whip together the yogurt, orange blossom water, vanilla and 1 tablespoon (15 ml) of honey in a bowl until smooth and light and garnish with fresh orange zest. You can easily use a fork and small bowl to whip it up.

Serve the mini tarts with a dollop of orange blossom yogurt.

 TIP: Use a fork to make small indents in the middle of the mini tarts, which will help the edges rise, forming a border.

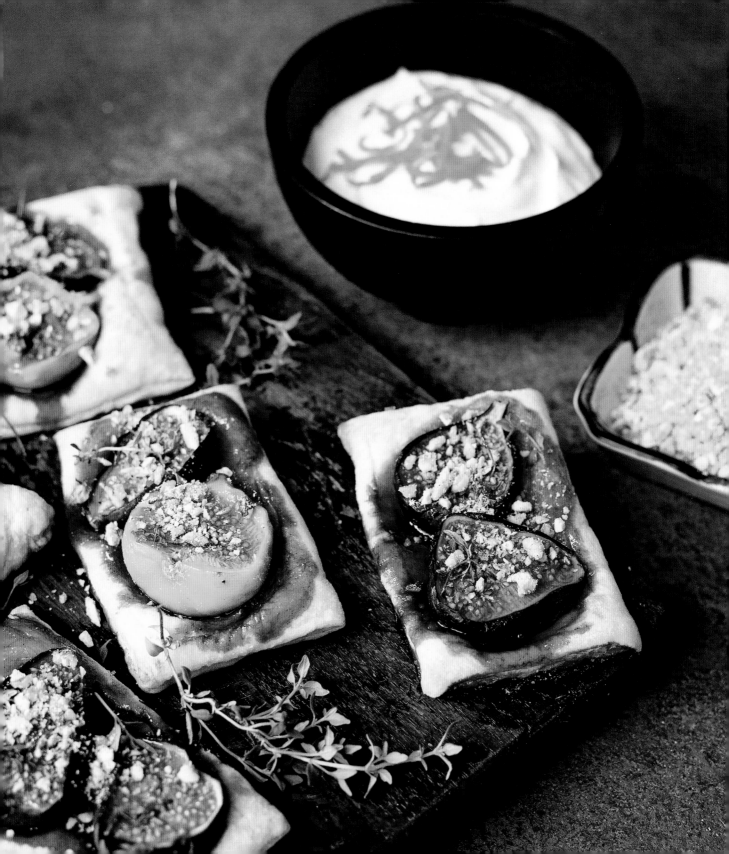

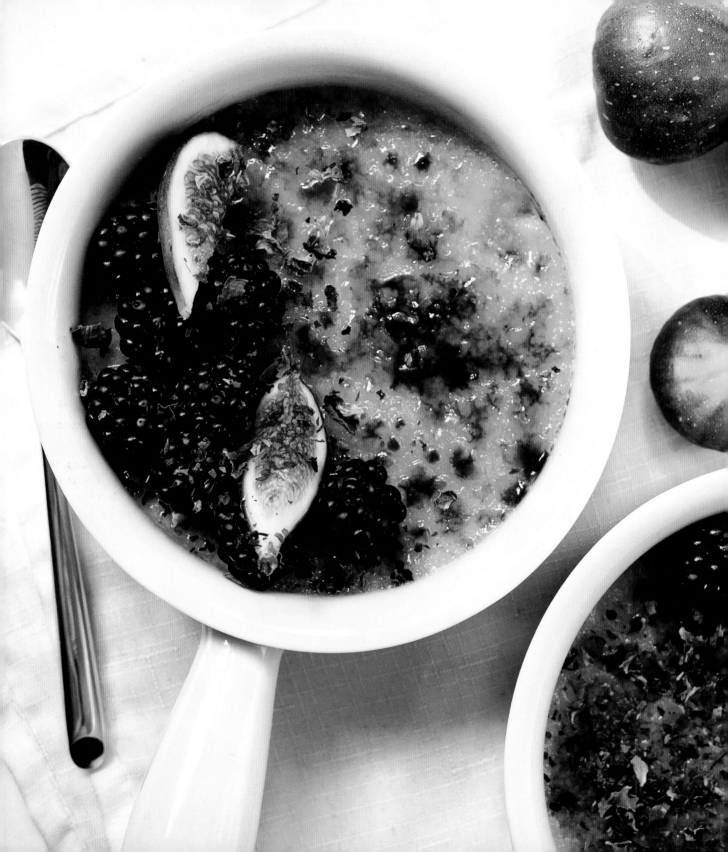

ROSE-SAFFRON CRÈME BRÛLÉE

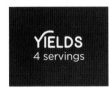

YIELDS
4 servings

There are a few indulgences I lust after, and the initial crack of the carmelized sugar on crème brûlée is one of them. Steeped with saffron threads and a drop of rose water, these crème brûlées are aromatic and perfumed with a brilliant Persian flair.

The beautiful thing about crème brûlée is that you can make them ahead of time, and then brûlée the sugar right before serving.

1½ cups (360 ml) heavy cream

½ cup (120 ml) whole milk

¼ tsp saffron threads

1 tsp extract, vanilla paste or
1 vanilla bean

⅓ cup (66 g) sugar, plus more for
brûlée crust

6 egg yolks

1 tbsp (15 ml) rose water

Hot water

Dried rose petals, for garnish

Fruit, for garnish

Preheat the oven to 325°F (163°C).

In a pot, heat together the heavy cream, milk, saffron and vanilla. If using a vanilla bean, cut it down the center and scrape out the seeds and add both the seeds and bean to the milk mixture.

Bring to a gentle boil and then allow to cool for 10 minutes. Discard the vanilla bean.

In another bowl, whisk together the sugar, egg yolks and rose water. Slowly stream the egg mixture into the milk mixture while whisking until fully incorporated. Be sure not to add all at once as you may scramble the eggs. If you do see some scrambled pieces, strain the mixture through a sieve.

Place four 6-ounce (180-ml) ramekins in a roasting pan (or cake pan) and pour the cream mixture into the ramekins. Pour enough hot water into the roasting pan to come up halfway on the ramekins.

Bake for about 40 minutes until the custards are set and wiggle slightly. Once done, remove from the oven and refrigerate for at least 2 hours. When ready to serve, sprinkle enough sugar to lightly coat the top in an even layer. Use a blowtorch or place under the broiler for a few minutes to brûlée the top until golden brown.

Top with rose petals and fresh fruit.

TAHINI DATE BITES WITH CARDAMOM

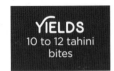

YIELDS
10 to 12 tahini bites

One of my favorite treats growing up was halvah, and it still is. Halvah is a creamy fudge-like sweet made from sesame paste with delicious Mediterranean fillings such as nuts and chocolate. Well, making halvah is a time-consuming process, and because we are all about quick and easy, these mini tahini bites provide the same creamy texture with healthy dates for sweetness, and nuts and seeds for crunch.

8 dried pitted dates, roughly chopped

5 dried apricots, roughly chopped

3 tbsp (45 ml) tahini

½ tsp ground cardamom

¼ cup (28 g) finely ground almonds

¼ cup (28 g) finely ground pistachios

¼ cup (36 g) toasted sesame seeds

¼ cup (15 g) dried rose petals

In a food processor, add the dates, apricots, tahini and cardamom and pulse until a well-combined thick mixture forms.

Wet your hands slightly and roll the mixture into 10 to 12 balls. Roll each ball into the nut, sesame seed or rose petal toppings.

Store in an airtight container in the refrigerator for up to 5 days.

 TIP: These tahini bites store incredibly well. Make a bigger batch and keep in the refrigerator in an airtight container for a quick, sweet, energizing bite.

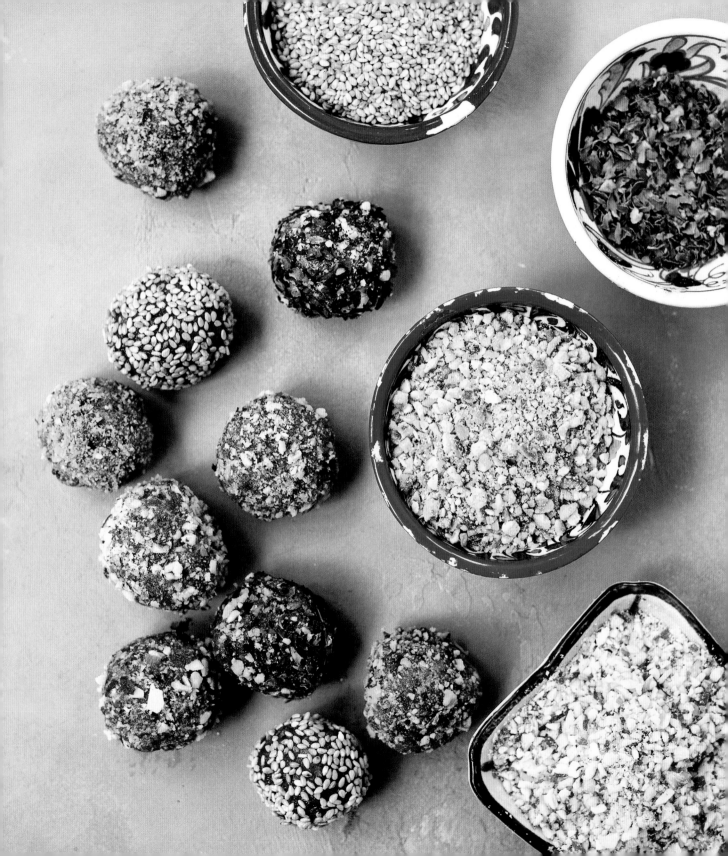

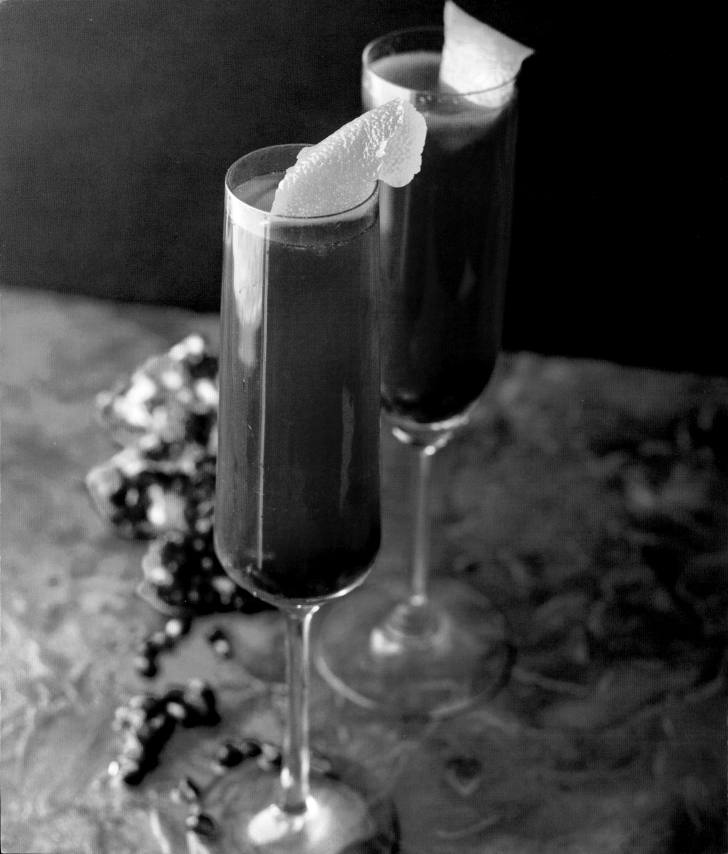

CITRUS POMEGRANATE COCKTAIL
with CARDAMOM

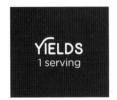

YIELDS
1 serving

A few years ago as we were walking the streets of Istanbul, we came across a local juice vendor who was squeezing fresh blood orange and pomegranate juice. The whiff of fresh citrus and the deep intoxicating color of pomegranate was addictive and striking, and the combination of flavors was just beautiful.

Here is a simple play on that memory. A small pinch of cardamom is added as a warm background note.

4 oz (120 ml) sparkling blood orange juice

½ oz (15 ml) gin or vodka

½ oz (15 ml) pomegranate juice

Pinch of ground cardamom

Ice for shaking

Strip of orange zest, using a vegetable peeler, for garnish

Pomegranate seeds, for garnish

Pour the blood orange juice into a tall champagne glass. In a shaker, add the gin, pomegranate juice and a pinch of cardamom with ice. Shake and strain into the glass. Garnish with the orange peel and pomegranate seeds.

 TIP: If you can find sparkling blood orange juice, by all means use that, but any sparkling citrus juice will work for this.

MUDDLED MINT AND CUCUMBER COOLER

YIELDS
1 serving

There is nothing cooler on a summer's day than this cucumber cooler. Inspired by the popular Israeli cocktail limonana, I took the flavors of mint and lemon and made an oh-so-easy cocktail that you can whip up any night of the week.

5–6 slices cucumber, plus more for garnish

¼ cup (5 g) fresh mint leaves, plus more for garnish

1 cup (240 ml) lemonade

1 oz (30 ml) gin or vodka

Muddle 3 to 4 slices of cucumber with the mint in a shaker with ice, lemonade and gin. Shake well and pour into a tall 8-ounce (240-ml) glass. Garnish with extra cucumber slices and mint leaves.

 TIP: This can easily be made into a "mocktail." Just omit the alcohol and substitute with sparkling water.

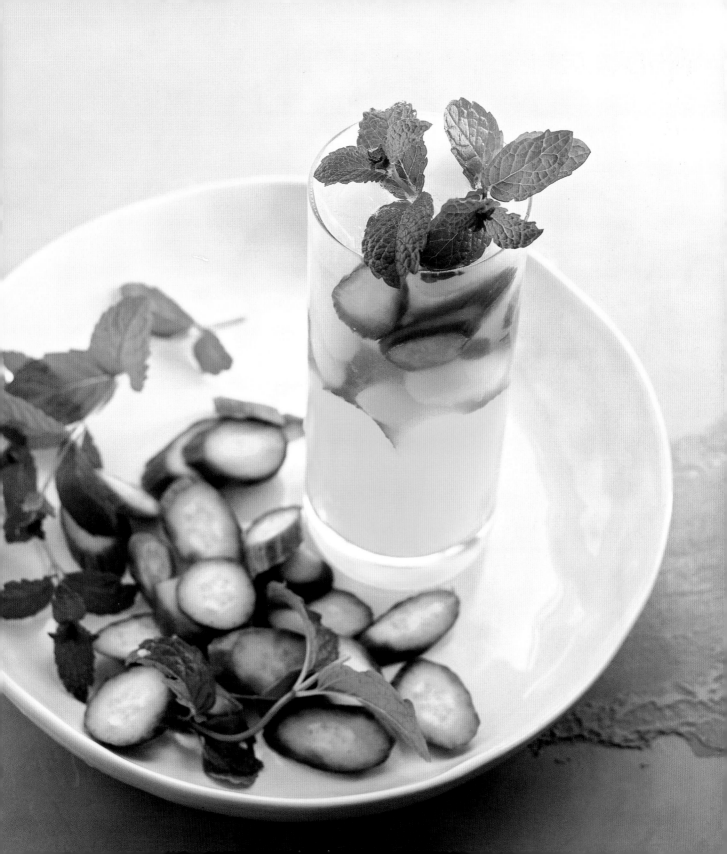

ACKNOWLEDGEMENTS

This wouldn't be a dream come true without the support system I have—small but mighty! There are no words to express how thankful I am.

My best friend of almost 20 years, you and I have been through a lot together, and I am so thankful for our ongoing friendship. Dominee, you are more like a sister than a friend, and I am so thankful for our friendship. Thank you for being my confidant and schlepping all the way here to help me recipe test during the summer. We had fun!

I have some amazing and powerful women in my life that I have known for a while, and new friends that have become very special to me. Jeana, Katie, Ashley C. and Rosanna—you ladies are not just girlfriends, but are like my sisters. I miss you and am thankful you are part of my life.

To my mom, who initially instilled culture in me, dragging me to musicals and plays when I was little and forcing me to roll grape leaves and appreciate foods and flavors for as long as I can remember. I think I got the creative gene from you, so thank you, Mom, and I love you!

My mother-in-law, Deb, I hope you know how special you are to me. Thank you for being a beam of wisdom and class, and for tasting anything I put in front of you with a generous smile and willing palate.

To my blog friends Shannon S., Shanna S., Miriam, P. and Amy K. You all are inspiring and motivating, and I am so thankful to have you all to lean on. You have become more than internet acquaintances. You are the professional, funny and smart women that I admire and respect.

To my trusted and hungry blog readers. I still remember the day I had a handful of readers (that weren't my family) and the first comment I received. I am so thankful for every single person that reads my site, cooks and shares their family recipe traditions. Thank you for being a part of this journey.

Thank you to all the generous recipe testers: Jessica H., Heather E., Shana D., Caryn S., Amber D., Karla D., Kate B., Deb E., Corrina H., Natalie G., Nicole K., Natasha K., Alyssa B., Chris L., Samantha A., Scott G., Emma U. and Katie S. Your feedback means a lot to me, and I appreciate everything you did. Thank you!

To the team at Page Street who saw something in me and my passion, and created something amazing, thank you! Thank you to my editor, Sarah, for your undeniable patience and professionalism, which I value so much. Thank you for your guidance.

Last but never the least, I wanted to dedicate the last few words to my best friend, my partner in life and my husband, Joe. I am so blessed and thankful beyond belief to have you by my side. You have been nothing but supportive, loving and encouraging, and none of this would have happened without the unconditional love and respect I get from you. I love you and Hula more than words can express, and I love our little family.

ABOUT THE AUTHOR

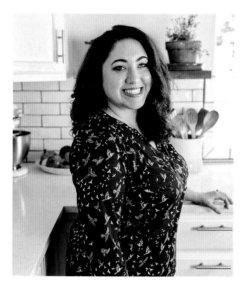

Samantha Ferraro is the blogger and creator of the food blog, The Little Ferraro Kitchen, where she shares world cuisine recipes, spanning different cultures and ethnicities.

Her recipes have been shared with the *LA Times*, *Huffington Post* and *Cosmopolitan*, and she is a regular contributor for other online publications. Samantha has lived in several major areas, including New York City, Hawaii, California and the Pacific Northwest, illustrating her diverse knowledge of culture and food.

When Samantha isn't in the kitchen, she is out enjoying the beauty of the Pacific Northwest with her husband Joe and their dog Hula in Bellingham, Washington.

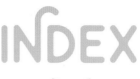

INDEX